MW00932653

HEALTHY BODY

Twelve Principles for Peace, Health and Crazy Joy

Dr. DiAnna Wallace, N.D.

Naturopathic Doctor

Dedication

This book was ready to be published on June 22, 2017. But my husband Tim had begun to feel fatigue and weakness about a month before that, so I decided to wait until he got to feeling better before I published it and its forthcoming companion products.

In July, 2017, Tim was diagnosed with a rare and aggressive form of cancer. He fought a brave and relentless battle with this merciless disease before retiring his body and graduating to heaven in March, 2018. While he never got to read this finished book, nor even its manuscript, he lived many of the principles within. He enthusiastically encouraged my personally adopting the principles I'll share with you. He witnessed the transformation in my life. And he was supportive of my sharing my story and these life-changing habits through this work.

He was one of my guinea-pigs during my early natural health education. He was my best friend. He was a constant source of deep-belly laughter and inspiration. He was the kind of dad every daughter wishes she could have. He loved his Father God, and he loved me well for over thirty years. He finished well. And yet, even in his absence my life has gone on.

The book you hold in your hands is one of the projects that kept me going during the season of his illness and the season since. I believe this project is part of my divine purpose and an assignment on my life. I began writing it in March 2012. For over seven years it has taken on different forms. First it was a small group study. Then its subjects were delivered through talks to various women's groups. Later it became an online group coaching program, and now, finally, as a book that will be followed up with a Journal for Your Journey, then a devotional book.

I would like to thank so many other people in addition to Tim who have contributed to this project. My daughter Bailey has encouraged me to continue this work. I've seen her incorporate many, if not all of these principles over the past several years. She has celebrated many small milestones along the way to publication. My sisters DeNisha McCollum, DeMarie Patterson, and Debi Hale have been constant sources of encouragement. Their families have cheered me on, too! For the past couple years, Chrissie Doyle, has prodded me to hurry up and get this thing published. Trudy Bonnette has been with me since my first trip to Alaska when I attended the Wellspring School of Ministry. Rick Bonnette was my carpool partner during the two-week school. He helped me process much of this new-found freedom that I'm eager to share with you. Becky Harmon helped me during the re-writing process in 2015. I remember her telling me my first manuscript was "too clinical." And she was right! If you think the first two chapters are "clinical" now, you should have seen them before Becky got a hold of me! Heidi Colligan has served as a midwife for getting this "baby" delivered. She has held my hand (even though we've yet to meet in person) and walked me through the final stages of birthing this book.

I'm blessed with many supportive people in my life. The past couple of years have been surreal and I could not have emerged from such an unforeseen season without their prayers and words of encouragement.

But it is my desire to dedicate this book to you, the reader. It's my prayer that each page will prickle your heart with hope for better, better health, better relationships with your family and friends, a better relationship with yourself, and especially a deeper relationship with our Father God who loves you so extravagantly every single day in ways you may not be aware of now. It's my hope that you will begin to see His love for you in a bigger way. As you release the pains from your past, as you begin to make changes to your food selections and physical habits, it's my prayer that you will become more of a conduit that is able to allow His love flow through you more freely, without getting snagged on the hurts that may have held you back in the past. You have so much to look forward to. And I've prayed for you for years, that this little yellow book in your hands will be a power tool to help you Heal Thy Body. I love you. And I pray God's very best for you!

Table of Contents

Introduction... 1

Chapter One: Your Food Affects Your Mood: 6

Chapter Two: Toxins are Everywhere............................. 26

Chapter Three: Your Body is a Temple – Keep it Clean............... 42

Chapter Four: Walking is Good for Your Soul 56

Chapter Five: Forgiveness is a Gift You Give Yourself................ 66

Chapter Six: You are Wonderfully Made........................ 78

Chapter Seven: Choose to Speak Words of Life 92

Chapter Eight: Take Every Thought Captive 106

Chapter Nine: Fear Not.. 112

Chapter Ten: Play for an Audience of One 126

Chapter Eleven: Rejection is a Secret Saboteur 136

Chapter Twelve: Have a Happy Ending......................... 148

About DiAnna... 158

Introduction

The rest of your life can be the BEST of your life.

The book you hold in your hands has the power to transform your life in every area where you are feeling physical pain, hurt from your past, strains in your current relationships, and worries for your future. Sounds like a pretty tall order, doesn't it? You may wonder how I can say this.

The life-giving principles in Healthy Body are not just theories. Each and every principle you will discover has been tried and proven in my own life, and in the lives of hundreds of others with whom I've had the privilege to share over the past ten years.

What began as a personal journey to healing has grown into a tool of discovery, revelation, and hope for myself and others.

Healthy Body was birthed out of two purposes:

To Help Believers Break Through Spiritual Blocks to Healing

After practicing a few years as a Naturopathic Doctor, nutritionist, and herbalist, I noticed that while most of my clients experienced major improvements in the way they felt, some seemed to hit a wall and not continue to progress. Because I believe in the holistic nature of healing encompassing body, soul, and spirit, I suspected the wall may be spiritual in nature. I tried many solutions, but I just didn't know how to help these clients get the breakthrough they needed for further healing.

As a pastor's wife and active church member for over 20 years, I had often wondered why people in the church were just as sick as those who weren't. Why were so many people in our congregations dealing with health challenges when we have access to the healing power of Jesus Christ? I knew that that some of those illnesses were related to lifestyle choices, but there had to be something more. My search for healing led me to the Wellspring School of Ministry in Anchorage, Alaska, and it was there that I really began to understand healing on a spiritual level. The second purpose for the Healthy Body Book is:

To Bring Physical and Spiritual Healing to the Body of Christ

I believe that as members of the Body of Christ begin to implement the principles of nutrition, fitness, forgiveness, and dealing with spiritual strongholds; not only will individuals be restored to health, but healing will spread throughout HIS body, the church.

The title of this book, *Healthy Body* is a play on words. Not only will incorporating the principles in this book lead to a healthier physical body, they will help you **Heal-Thy-Body**. In Ephesians 4:16

we read, "He makes the whole body fit together perfectly. As each part does its own special work, it helps the other parts grow, so that the whole body is healthy and growing and full of love." (The Living Bible) The whole body can't really be healthy and full of love if it is hurting from a painful past, or making unhealthy lifestyle choices can it?

The Healthy Body system uniquely integrates principles that impact the individual's health and well-being which will contribute to the Body of Christ becoming healthier as these principles are learned, embraced, and practiced daily. Too many in the Church are struggling because of ignorance about natural laws concerning their physical health. Too many are struggling from broken relationships because they don't know how to finally forgive and receive relief from years of emotional hurt. Too many hurting people are hurting people, both inside and outside church walls with the unrecognized power of their spoken words. As these principles are learned and practiced daily, not only will the health of individuals improve, but it will spread hope and healing to the body of Christ.

While the first two chapters may sound a bit technical, we'll dig in to the good stuff right after, so don't get snaggled by the clinical terminology!

Are you ready to begin this new journey to your best health yet?

Some of the changes you will make as you read this book will be subtle, such as increasing the amount of water you drink so your body can release the toxic substances that have been sabotaging your health.

Oh sure, you may find yourself in the restroom a bit more frequently for a week or so, but would you rather have the toxic stuff inside or outside your body? Mmmhhhmmm, that's what I thought.

Some changes might be painful, like when you will dredge up memories from the past. This time we don't bring them up so we can talk about them then send them back to the recesses of our minds where they can continue to prickle us with pain, fear and even condemnation. No, this time is different. This time we bring them up for the purpose of doing the business necessary to deal with them and to rob them of the sting of pain they have too long inflicted into your life. There will be no more stuffing the pain from your past. When you dig in, do the work, and receive personal revelation, there will be no more pain. None. Really.

Some changes will require you to take a hard look at how you spend your time – how you prioritize yourself in your schedule – and carve out some time every single day to bless yourself. Sometimes we get blessings from other people. I believe God is always blessing us, we just don't always tune in to take notice. I believe He has given us the ability to bless ourselves through our thoughts, words, and actions. You are worth it! Don't freak out over this idea right now. Just let the seed of this idea fall on the fertile ground of your life. When the time comes, you'll discover creative ways to fit you (yes, even too-long-neglected **you**) back into your schedule. We'll talk about some simple, practical first steps to take to get you on the track to healing.

I'm excited to partner with you on this journey. No matter what your expectations, you have a lot to look forward to. There is freedom to discover and health to recover, and a whole new life of restored, redeemed and healthy relationships to look forward to.

Now, let's get started healing YOUR body!

Chapter One

Your Food Affects Your Mood

Have you ever thought about the possibility that the food we eat affects and defines, our body's ability to function and heal?

The bottom line is that what you eat affects how you feel. This is even more important than whether or not your joints ache, your stomach hurts, or your running time needs to be faster. What you eat has a tremendous influence over your mental processes such as clear thinking, managing frustrations, and your ability to practice self-control. Can you see how these factors affect not only you, but also your relationships with the people around you? We are going to spend the majority of this first chapter covering some basics about nutrition. I know, you may be thinking, "I thought this was a spiritual course." Well, let me ask you this sassy question: "Just where do you think the Holy Spirit is living these days?"

Far beyond all the other amazing functions your body performs on a daily basis, and most impressively, your body serves as a temple of the Holy Spirit of the Most High God. Think about it this way: How well will you serve others for the Kingdom after you have died? While no one knows exactly when his hour to die will be, there are some non-negotiable laws set in place in nature that affect how long we are likely to live. And the quality of our life while we are still alive is based largely on our daily food choices. If we prematurely abbreviate our lives by frequent poor food choices, not only will we be hard to be around – we will miss out on fulfilling the purposes for which we are created. I don't want to miss out on that, and I know you don't want to either!

People are deceived when they believe that their lifestyle, food, and health choices today don't really matter. There is a lack of connection between what we eat, what we do and how we feel. I have actually heard someone say during a class I was teaching that the FDA wouldn't pass foods that were bad for us! Why then do many drugs have deathly side effects, many of the foods in your local grocery store and fast food restaurants do as well, and the affect is cumulative over time. There's an old saying, that if you eat the "foods" from a box, you will end up in a box – much sooner. People don't have to die this way! There are better options . . . interestingly from God's Creation. We are generally healthier when we eat foods as closely as possible to how they occur in nature. For example, fresh vegetables are a rockin' blessing to our bodies. They are chock full of nutrition and deliciousness!

As it turns out, you can only serve God's purposes for you on this earth as long as you are alive. Let that sink in. Once we die, we can no longer serve others here on earth for the Kingdom of God.

Suddenly, the proper care and feeding of our body becomes a significant stewardship issue. It's important. It's essential. And it is so easy to neglect or even abuse. As you continue through this book, you will be empowered to make healthier choices that will create a healthier home for the Holy Spirit in your body.

You know, when you're born, your body arrives complete with all-new custom-engineered parts, adaptive capabilities like no other creation, self-regulating systems including blood pressure, breathing, regular sleep patterns, digestion, and an immune system to fight off illness. It includes a handsome or beautiful custom face (even if it does resemble your Aunt Martha on your dad's side!). Your body performs more important and complex functions that any vehicle, computer, or other man-made creation.

Our bodies are designed to serve us for about a hundred years. Doesn't it seem possible we take our body's reliability for granted? Sure we do! Most Americans consume what's known as the "Standard American Diet." Do you notice the initials for this diet, S.A.D.? That pretty much sums it up. It's tragic that we are more interested in convenience than in quality. Our family meals are too often consumed in the car while driving 75 miles per hour down the highway, music or movies playing, while we bite, chomp, chomp, gulp. Does that sound familiar to you? Seriously, *eating while driving is a crime we commit against our bodies.* When we are driving, healthful eating flies out the window, so to speak, the moment we roll down our window to place an order at the drive through.

Some national restaurant chains have made intentional efforts to improve their offerings, but the menu at most drive-thru establishments consists of foods designed to be eaten conveniently and quickly. They are usually pretty easy to hold in one hand while driving with the other, right? We know that foods in the convenience category are generally sandwiches, breaded chicken, French fries, soft drinks, and possibly a fried pie or brownie for dessert. Really? Where is the nutrition in that? So, everyone in the family orders their favorite meal by number, and then they are off and running again in no time.

In our convenience-based world, there seems to be too little time for planning and preparing meals that are rich in nutrition and taste. And what about the old-fashioned concept of families sitting around a table at the end of the day eating nutritious and delicious food? Oh sure, it happens in a few families, but not many, and not often. Did you know your stomach actually needs a quiet, peaceful setting to do its best digestion work?

Flying down the highway just does not lend itself to great digestion. You don't chew your food as many times, and it is seldom a peaceful, calm environment due either to traffic outside, or some kind of family tension inside the fast-moving vehicle. And while a peaceful dinner with the family around the table may seem like more work than it is worth, it does lend itself to not only improved digestion, but also improved relationships. Does that sound worth it to you?

Just how big a deal is it that we make healthy food choices? Does it really make a difference if we make a decision to upgrade our fuel?

You bet it does! Let's take a moment to see where you currently are in the dietary selection department. Are you average? Above average? Or below average? For example:

Each year, the *average* American consumes:

176 pounds of sugar

120 orders of French fries

150 slices of pizza

190 candy bars

In this instance, I hope you are below average! Eating this way only creates deficiencies in your body that lead to break downs, some emotional, some physical, some relational. Yes, the food you eat affects your mood.

As a nutritionist, I have taught classes on how participants can upgrade their food choices in order to better manage their weight. Usually in about the third week of a class series, someone will pipe up and say they have noticed that they can either think more clearly, and their mood is significantly improved, or both. They ask if it is possible that this may be related to their change in diet? Others in the group invariably chime in that they are experiencing the same thing. It's always one of those "Glory Hallelujah!" moments for me, because it shows me, and them, and the others in the class that they have made the connection between mood and food.

Good food makes for a good mood.

Once this connection is established, it will be with them for the rest of their lives. They will continue to make great choices throughout the duration of the class, then as time goes on afterward, they may tend to venture back into the land of old habits. They are not off course for long before mood swings, irritability, temper flares, feelings of depression, nervousness, or anxiety rear their ugly heads. Oh, maybe my class participant doesn't notice it first, maybe a family member points it out to them (ouch!) and they have an opportunity to get back on track.

Am I suggesting that all mood swings, temper flares, depression, feelings of nervousness, anxiety and irritability are caused by diet? Yes, I am saying that diet affects all of these. Improving your daily food choices can and will affect each of them for your life, too. Conversely, if we're already in a bad mood, it's more likely we will make a "bad" food choice, right? Most people have experienced this vicious cycle. Sometimes it's a "once in a blue moon" experience, but for many, it's a several-times-a-day emotional eating roller coaster.

Let's take a few minutes to break it down and see just how different kinds of food can affect our mood.

There are three main components to food. Understanding a bit about what each of them "brings to the table" helps us be more intentional when we are preparing to order something to eat at a restaurant, or while we are grocery shopping for our family. The three main parts of food are: Proteins, Carbohydrates, and Fats. Let's look at the benefit each of these brings to our body. This information may be a reminder you, or it may seem like we are revisiting your high school Biology class. Here's the perk, this time it will make more sense! You may even begin to realize that class wasn't a waste of time in the first place.

Proteins

While each of the food categories is essential to helping our body operate at its best, *protein is the most important,* and most people don't get enough protein in their daily diet. What makes protein so special? It provides essential amino acids for our tissues to be able to heal and repair themselves. Now, any time you hear the word "essential" when it comes to nutrition, it means that it's *essential* to get that nutrient from your diet because the body can't manufacture it itself. So, these essential amino acids are necessary for the body to maintain important muscle mass and you must get them from your diet as your body can't manufacture them on its own.

Maintaining muscle mass is especially important as we age. Beginning around age 40, we lose muscle mass each year, unless we are intentional about maintaining it. Muscle is important for many reasons. It helps keep our bones strong by providing tension on them. Muscle burns more calories than fat, so if we let our muscle mass decrease, we may still see the same weight on the scales at age 40 that we did at 25, but we don't wear the same size clothes and our body looks more lumpy and bumpy than it did back then, too! This happens because even though the scales haven't changed, our body composition has. By increasing protein consumption, and adding weight or resistance training, muscle mass can be maintained, and even gained.

Have you noticed that most people get shorter as they age? This is due to their losing muscle tone. Healthy, strong muscles are responsible for supporting the skeletal system. When the muscles no longer get enough protein, or if the digestive system can't efficiently process the protein the body takes in, the muscles lose mass. As muscle mass declines, the person begins to get shorter and usually begins to slump over. That slumping creates a whole gaggle of issues for the internal organs that begin to experience weight and pressure they were never designed to withstand. The body literally begins to cave in on itself as posture worsens.

Keep in mind this important fact about your body: ***God made your body to heal itself***. It is constantly in the process of healing and repairing itself. If you are off track on your health, **today** is always the best day to start taking steps to renew it. Your body is forgiving. Making a few changes will allow your good health to return.

On our plates, protein looks like eggs, chicken, beef, fish, milk, cottage cheese, cheese, yogurt, and legumes (beans such as pintos, chickpeas, and lentils.)

Consider beginning your day with a couple of eggs. This helps keep blood sugar stable all day long and will help you manage your appetite throughout the day, plus they are protein-rich little powerhouses and great for your brain, too! Don't be concerned about the possible cholesterol in eggs. Here's something few people realize about the incredible egg: the yolk is mostly fat, the white is mostly protein, and rich in lecithin. Lecithin is a natural emulsifier of fat. It breaks down the fats in the yolk so your body can use them. How cool is that? God provides for us in so many ways, and I'm always intrigued to discover these kinds of things as I study nutrition.

If you can't eat or don't like eggs, consider a protein supplement product and shoot for getting 30 grams of protein within 30 minutes of waking. This is a quick, efficient way to replenish amino acids that have been burned off by your body's self-cleaning processes as you slept the night before. Many people who begin the simple practice of getting 30 grams of protein within 30 minutes of waking report more sustained energy throughout the entire day, fewer blood sugar fluctuations, and other improvements in the way their body functions overall.

Including protein in every meal and with each snack is a good way to maintain muscle mass, promote healing, growth in children, and to keep your blood sugar stable. Having boiled eggs on hand or quickly mixing up a shaker cup with protein powder are two easy ways to be sure you are getting enough protein to support your healthy body every day.

Sugar

Alright, let's move on to the most common simple carbohydrate and the ultimate anti-nutrient so readily available in our diets today:

sugar. I'd like to take a few minutes to share with you about my personal relationship with sugar.

I never had much of a "sweet tooth" but one of my younger sisters was THE sweet tooth in our family. She loved candy! Any time we were near any kind of candy, it was like she could smell it. Then she would "sniff it out" to find it and ask if she could have it. I usually wasn't interested in candy much. I first noticed a sensitivity to sugar when I was very young. Every time I ate cotton candy at the county fair, I threw it up. In in fifth grade (yes, I still remember where I was and how it all went down, or came up as the case may have been). I had just eaten the last popsicle I ever would because I threw it up about five minutes later, yet somehow I did not realize I had a sugar issue!

Fast forward several years. When I was twenty-three, I began to have sugar "episodes" that went something like this. I would have something with sugar in it, (it didn't even have to be candy, cake, or particularly rich.) It just needed to contain sugar as an ingredient and within thirty minutes I would be super-hyper; often singing and being absolutely intoxicated for a few minutes. Then it felt like the top of my head flew off and my hands and feet would go numb then I would fall into a deep sleep for about 20 hours! Upon awakening, I could look forward to a big fat headache for three days. My husband literally carried me into the house on many occasions after I crashed and he could not wake me up. You are probably wondering, did I go to the doctor? Sure I did! I had a glucose tolerance test during which I felt like I was going to flip off the table, I saw things that were not there, I chilled, I slept, and I felt completely insane. And guess what? In spite of all that, my blood sugar levels were "within normal limits".

There was nothing "wrong" with me. So, my doctor told me to avoid sugar since it seemed my body didn't know what to do with it. I kid you not, I paid a lot of money for confirmation of the very thing that had become painfully obvious to me. I could not tolerate sugar in any form in any food. So, I stopped eating all sugar-containing foods. That included not only the obvious, but even salad dressings, ketchup, baked beans, cereals, most rolls, and the list went on. As long as I stayed away from sugar, I felt better. It seemed to me like my food options became really sparse. So, if you can't eat sugar, where do you turn to for sweetening options? Enter Aspartame, or NutraSweet as I almost-lovingly called it. Oh yes, those glorious little blue packets "saved my life", or so I thought. Since I didn't want to feel any deprived from this new dietary restriction, and being the creative person I am, I simply learned to duplicate any sugar-containing food using artificial sweetener! Sounds harmless enough, right?

Within a couple years, I began to experience significant vision decline. Every six months, my vision prescription changed as my vision worsened. This continued for about seven years. My eye doctor asked if I had blood sugar issues. I technically didn't, but we couldn't find another reason for the vision loss. Then I learned about the damaging effects of aspartame on the nerves. I knew the optic nerve was a nerve (yes, I know, brilliant revelation there and I hadn't even started my natural health studies, yet!). I then made the painful decision to eliminate my "crutch" from my diet. At the same time I began to supplement with some vitamins and antioxidants to see if that would help.

Within six weeks I no longer needed my glasses to see to drive during the day. Within about three months I didn't need them at night, either. My vision returned completely! I could once again see "like a hawk" without glasses or contacts. Did I have powerful withdrawal headaches from the artificial sweeteners? YES! But it was so worth it! And I didn't die from not having sweet foods! I learned to cook with honey and continued to live without sugar, for a total of 19 years. I'll share my story of healing from the sugar issue when we get into a later chapter, but even today, I don't eat much sugar. As you will see, it does far too much damage to our body, but not more damage than artificial sweeteners, and there are no real benefits except for what happens on the tip of the tongue. Oh, the many ways our tongue can get us into trouble! We'll discover more about the destructive power of the tongue in a later chapter.

Sugar is a tricky "food" because it doesn't contain any nutrients. As if being totally void of any nutrition weren't "bad" enough, it still requires nutrients to be processed in the body. So, if you eat a piece of candy, cake, drink a soda, or any other way to consume sugar. Your body is tasked with finding nutrients to process that sugar. If you don't take in food with some kind of nutrition at the same time, your body will have to rob nutrients from its own stores to process that sugar. As it uses nutrients from its own stores, *your immune system is compromised for about 30 minutes after consuming a sugary snack.*

Have you ever noticed that cold and flu season follows Halloween, Christmas, and Valentine's Day? It's really no wonder with all that candy sugar flowing through our bloodstreams!

Consuming sugar also leads to inflammation in the body. Some have suggested that sugar is inflammation's favorite food! Inflammation is a root issue for aging, heart disease, diabetes, Alzheimer's, and other issues. In fact, recent studies are calling Alzheimer's Type 3 diabetes. What if it's really all about a body's inability to process sugars? Reducing sugar consumption reduces inflammation. Most of my clients notice that their joints don't ache as much (or at all) during a sugar-free cleansing program that I recommend. Consider accepting a 30-day (or longer) no-sugar challenge yourself. The first three or four days are the most challenging, then you will notice a fresh mental clarity, renewed energy, and who knows what other perks!

Sugar in our diet suppresses the release of Human Growth Hormone (HGH), so we start noticing more wrinkles, skin spots, fat accumulation, and other age-related issues if we continue to consume it.

And sugar in the diet raises insulin levels. This is a natural response in the body to manage the levels of sugar in the bloodstream. If there is too much sugar, the pancreas will secrete insulin to balance the blood sugar levels. If we continue to abuse our body with sugary foods, we create too much stress on the pancreas for it to keep up with blood sugar spikes from meals that are too big and sugar-laden snacks and desserts. We may need to supplement with additional insulin to keep our blood sugar in check. This is known as diabetes. Type II Diabetes is a lifestyle disease that can usually be prevented by lifestyle choices or corrected by lifestyle changes. I'm not saying it is easy, but I am saying it can be done. If you are willing to make some short-term uncomfortable changes for some long-term benefits, you can expect to live healthier for a longer time.

Does this mean you have to completely eliminate all forms of sugar from your diet? It can be done as I can personally attest, and it leads to slower aging, improved immune function, less inflammation, less pain, and an overall sense of improved well-being. However, if that seems just a bit too extreme for your preferences, then the next question might be, is there a good time to have sugar?

After a vigorous workout, your cells can more efficiently use sugar in the bloodstream, which then requires less insulin. It may actually promote quicker recovery when paired with protein. So, once you've put in a *vigorous* workout, enjoying a little sugar/protein combo might not be a bad idea. Otherwise, keep in mind that sugar truly does nothing FOR your body, but it can certainly HARM it in many ways.

The second type of carbohydrates is **Complex.** Complex carbs are digested more slowly than simple carbohydrates since they contain fiber. The body has to work harder and longer to break down fiber in foods. The presence of fiber in a food slows the release of sugar into the bloodstream. This is a good thing. When the sugar enters the bloodstream more slowly, we are less likely to experience "spikes" in blood sugar, or brief episodes of hyperactivity followed by the "after-crash". Complex carbs also contain nutrients (vitamins, minerals, and even some healthy fats) and are definitely the more healthy option of the two types of carbs. Some examples of complex carbohydrates ar vegetables, fruits, whole grains, nuts, and seeds.

Some people think eating complex carbs takes more time to prepare and consume than simple carbs. And while it is true that these foods do require more time chewing them properly before swallowing, I think bananas, apples, pears, peaches, carrots, cherry tomatoes were the original fast foods, and the list goes on.

Of all the food types, taking the time to chew your food is especially important for proper digestion of carbs. Carbohydrate digestion begins in the mouth. There are enzymes in your saliva that begin to break down the carbohydrates into sugars that your body can use. If we do not take the time to chew our carbs, they move on down the digestive tract undigested. If the liver does not produce the enzymes needed to break them down, the pancreas can make those enzymes.

I think of it like this, the pancreas has a full-time job managing your blood sugar levels and secreting insulin as necessary to keep blood sugar levels in a healthy range and it can also "moonlight" as an enzyme generator when necessary. But, when we eat extra-large portions or too many sugary foods, the pancreas must spend more time at its "part time job" and over time, it can just wear out. Taking time to chew your food, (at least 15 to 20 times each bite, especially for carbs) is important for proper digestion and to keep your pancreas from having to "moonlight" to the point of exhaustion. While it may take a while to adjust to chewing your food this many times, and heaven knows it impairs mealtime conversation during this "training period", after a while, you won't even think about it. You'll automatically know the feeling of the consistency of the food before you swallow it. Ideally, chewed food should be about the consistency of cake batter before going down the esophagus.

Carbohydrates

Too often, carbohydrates (carbs) get a bad rap. Carbohydrates in the diet are essential for energy. We need them in our diet so our body will have the fuel to carry out all the many jobs it has. Adequate energy at the cellular level is necessary for cells to take in nutrients and get rid of toxins. Every organ and gland must have enough energy to perform its unique task to keep us upright and running. We all know the feeling of not having enough energy to do all the great things we want to do! That's no fun! Our body gets most of its energy from carbohydrates, BUT . . . . and this is a big BUT. . .

Not All Carbs Are Created Equal

There are two types of carbohydrates: **Simple and Complex**.

Simple carbs are quickly and easily broken down into sugar for the body to use for energy. That sounds good, right? But it isn't really good at all. The main reason they are broken down simply is that they contain very little fiber and hardly any nutrients. So when they are consumed our bloodstream is quickly flooded with sugar. Oh sure, that is all fun and games, for about 25 minutes, then we either "need" some more, or we crash. No fun for us and no fun for the people around us as our blood sugar spikes then crashes! Some examples of simple carbs include: donuts, cake, candy, cookies, brownies, pastas, French fries, potato chips, most breads and crackers. You get the idea, common "junk" foods!

The effect these foods have on our mood is important to consider. While some people are more sensitive to fluctuations in their blood sugar levels than others, everyone is affected by these kinds of foods that crash after the sugar has quickly entered and then left our bloodstream. This leads to a feeling of let-down and we may notice it is harder to think clearly. Often, we will notice that those around us become irritable or more easily agitated during this crash time. (Of course we don't notice this in ourselves, it has to be *their* issue, right?)

Fats (Lipids)

The next food category is fats. Like carbs, fats have been scorned and excluded from too many diets. Old-school thinking was that fats made you fat. But would you like to know what really makes someone fat? Unnecessary sugars, poorly digested (unchewed) carbohydrates, unhealthy fats, lack of physical activity and excessive portion sizes are what lead to excess fat. Eliminating or strictly reducing healthy fats just leads to poor brain function, wacky hormones, stressed out nerves, hair loss, shaking, and the list goes on. How big a deal is that?

Like carbs, there are different kinds of fats. Let's take a moment to look at some examples of healthy fats first. These come from natural sources. They are not hydrogenated, preferably unrefined, nor otherwise "improved upon" by man. Think olive oil, coconut oil, nuts, flax seeds (freshly ground), fish, avocadoes, and olives.

The body uses these nutrient-dense fats to support our brain (which is about 70% fat in dry weight), our nerves, and our skin. Beneath our skin, fats help the walls of our cells, arteries, and veins remain pliable. We want our blood vessels to remain pliable like a blade of grass that bends easily. Over time, consuming "bad" fats, or not enough good fats can cause our blood vessels to lose pliability and become more like a garden hose that is rigid. Fats help these super important body parts remain pliable so they can do their jobs. (I can't pass up this opportunity to share that studies have shown that unaddressed anger, hostility, and frustration can also result in more rigid blood vessels and high blood pressure.) As we work through the processes of forgiving others and ourselves most often the anger issues that used to torment us will disappear.

Low-fat or no-fat diets are actually dangerous to the overall function of the body. Fats are necessary for proper hormone production, too. When there's not enough fat in the diet, hormonal cycles, and balances get off kilter. The skin becomes dry, wrinkled, or shriveled. Hair may begin to fall out. I don't know if you have ever had a known hormone imbalance, or if you have been around someone who does, but it can be stressful for the person with the situation, AND the people around them. There are usually mood swings with verbal outbursts, but feeling anxious and depressed are also common symptoms. Including at least some healthy fat in your daily diet will help prevent those kinds of stressors for you and for those you love!

Unhealthy fats include any fat that is hydrogenated or partially hydrogenated. If you see the word hydrogenated in the ingredients, put the box back on the shelf. The body can't process hydrogenated fats. They have been implicated in various diseases related to poor blood vessel health and it is best to avoid them like the plague. Focus on healthy fats in as natural, unrefined state as possible.

We've covered a lot of technical information in this chapter. I think of this first chapter as being nutrient dense with lots of valuable information not only what to eat – but why making healthier choices will result in a healthier body. While you won't have a test on this material, I hope you will keep it in mind as you make food selections in the coming week, months, and for the rest of your life. There is a strong connection between the food we eat and the mood we experience. Upgrade your food choices to whole foods, focus on healthy fats, proteins, and complex carbs. Avoid sugar and you will notice a marked improvement in your mood, energy level, and mental sharpness. This will likely cause reduction in various aches and pains. Like any other change, this may be uncomfortable at first, but it will be worth it - and you are worth the effort.

Chapter Two

Toxins are Everywhere

Let's talk about water. Since our body is over 70% water, and we can't manufacture water, we must drink it. Some people don't like water. "It's too boring," they say. Really? Let me ask you this, why do we not swim in the lake when it starts lightning? Because water is an excellent conductor of electricity. If we were in the lake and lightning struck, the water would quickly conduct the electrical current right to our body. We would be electrocuted and would likely die a "shocking" death. Surely that ability to conduct electricity is not boring. But yes, the taste can be a bit plain. Or you could think of it as a pure taste, not plain.

Do you realize your body is highly electric in nature? Have you ever taken someone to the hospital who thought they were having a heart attack? Within minutes of arriving, the person's chest is quickly dotted with several electrodes and the pattern of the electrical rhythm of his heart is recorded as an EKG (*electro*cardiogram). If someone is having stroke-like symptoms, an EEG (*electro*encephalogram) is recorded in a similar fashion, recording the electrical activity in the brain. But where does that electricity come from?

Nerve current produces constant electricity throughout the body. The head hosts the most electrical activity as the brain is constantly receiving and sending feedback from the rest of the body through the spinal cord and a complex network of nerves. The chest region hosts the second most electrical area (since the heart is an amazing muscle pumping from electrical impulses in the nervous system) and our hands and feet are surprisingly electrical as well. It is said that every nerve ends in either the hands or the feet. When you think about the sensitivity of our fingers and toes to temperatures, textures, and touch, it is obvious that there is a great deal of nerve activity there, but what makes that nerve activity possible is WATER. Water is the conductor for nerve activity in our body.

While the pure taste of water may seem dull or boring to some, it is important enough to be sure we are drinking it anyway. It is essential to so many functions in the body. Without adequate water intake, our body has to make life-altering decisions about what it will and will not be able to do. Yes, our body makes those decisions and we don't even have to have a single conscious thought about the matter. God literally wired us to live, but our "wires" need water to be able to do their job.

As if the nervous system weren't important enough, every single cell in your body requires plenty of water to receive nutrients from what we eat and more importantly, to be able to release toxins from the cell and have them literally washed out of our body. Without enough water, the cells become burdened with toxins, which leads to unhealthy cells. Unhealthy cells lead to unhealthy tissues. Unhealthy tissues lead to unhealthy organs. Unhealthy organs lead to unhealthy body systems. Unhealthy body systems lead to an unhealthy person! If you are not already drinking plenty of water, you will be amazed by how quickly you will notice improvements in your complexion, energy, elimination, and other important bodily functions.

How much water is enough? We read and hear that drinking 8 glasses of water a day is how much our body needs. So, let's think about that. Does it make sense to you that bigger bodies need more water than smaller bodies? After all, a bigger body has more cells to support and clean, so it makes sense that a bigger body needs more water than a smaller body. If you are drinking one to two glasses of water a day, you will definitely need to increase that amount, but just how much will be enough for your body?

A simple way to determine the optimal amount of water for you is this. Divide your body weight in half. The result is the ideal amount of ounces your body would like you to drink each day. For example, if you weigh 150 pounds, your ideal water consumption will be 75 ounces a day. BUT, if you are only drinking one or two glasses of water a day now, do not drink 75 ounces tomorrow! I've known people who hardly drank water at all then suddenly began to drink a lot of water. They got sick!

It's as if the whole body is suffering from dehydration until one day someone turns on a fire hose of water into it. Suddenly every cell is flooded with the water it needs to finally excrete toxins that have been hanging out in there far too long. I'm here to tell you, when an unusual amount of toxins hit your bloodstream at one time, for any reason, you will not feel well. A common example of this kind of rapid-onset toxicity is a hangover. The body's organs of elimination (lungs, liver, colon, lymph, and skin) are overwhelmed until they can work through the processes of eliminating the toxins. While a hangover is a result of higher levels of alcohol in the system, a similar effect may be felt if you finally give your body the water it needs and the cells begin to dump toxins into the bloodstream, but too much of a good thing isn't a good thing, right?

I suggest gradually increasing your water consumption rather than blasting your body with a bunch of water all at once. If you've been drinking two glasses of water a day, today drink three glasses. Tomorrow drink four glasses. The next day drink five glasses. You get the idea. Increase your water gradually.

A lot of people don't want to drink more water because they think it will make them go to the bathroom more frequently. Hmm, let's think about what happens when you go to the bathroom. Your body eliminates toxins from your body. You have a decision to make here. Would you rather have those toxins outside your body, or keep them inside your body? Of course you want those toxins out - but maybe you don't like the "every hour on the hour" bathroom visiting schedule? As you increase your water intake, your body will begin to play catch up. It will practically say to you, "THANK YOU!!! I can finally get some jobs done that I have had to put off because I didn't have enough water to get them done!" And, for a couple weeks or so, that will affect you in a "frequent flyer" (to the bathroom) kind of way. Keep in mind, the increase in frequency is a short-term side effect of increasing your water intake. Your body will quickly catch up and you will soon notice less frequent visits to the restroom.

A little note here. If you drink water at room temperature, you will likely notice less urgency to get to the restroom than if you drink it on ice. Plus, if it's already at room temperature when you drink it in, your body can put it right to work, rather than having to wait to bring it to body temperature before it can get into your bloodstream. Some people say that drinking it cold increases your metabolism because of the warming action required by the body. That may be the case, but you will have to decide if you prefer a faster metabolism that results in a faster trip to the loo, or a slower pace. Either way, taking steps to increase your water consumption is well worth any short-term inconvenience.

Water is Water

As we wrap up our discussion on water, keep in mind that water is water. Coffee is not water. Milk is not water. Soda pop is not water. Tea is not water. Water is water. While your body can extract water from water-rich foods like fruits and veggies, tea and coffee actually have a diuretic effect on the body. That means that even though they begin as water, the tea and coffee in them causes them to draw water out of the cells. I'm not suggesting you don't drink tea or coffee, just don't count them as water.

Toxins

One of the many benefits of drinking water is to help remove toxins from the cells and from the body. Toxins are substances that are not used to build the body's health. They are detrimental to the body in whole or in part. And they don't always leave the body in a timely manner. Some toxins may be stored in fat, bone, or muscle tissue and even wreak havoc on our health for years to come. But where do those toxins come from? Toxins are in our air, soil, water, food, clothing, body care products, medications, household cleaners, and too many other places to list here. In other words, toxins are all around us – pretty much everywhere we go.

Different toxins affect different parts of our bodies. Some have more effect on the nervous system (heavy metal toxicity). While others toxins affect the endocrine system, (think hormonal issues such as blood sugar regulation, menstrual irregularities, or infertility in men and women). It is well worth our effort to try to avoid the ones we can, knowing that there are too many to avoid them all. It is essential we take care of our body's elimination systems to give our bodies the best chance of getting rid of the toxins we can.

Here's the part where I call on your inner sleuth to begin a comprehensive investigation into the possible toxic chemicals lurking in your own home. They are all around from the kitchen, bathroom, living room, and even in the bedroom. You will soon become a master level label reader, and you will feel super empowered to know which toxins to look for and then kick them out! After all, you don't need that kind of negativity in your life, right?

Specific toxins to be on the lookout for and eliminate include:

Parabens

Parabens are commonly used preservatives in pharmaceutical and cosmetic products. They effectively prevent the growth of yeasts, molds, and bacteria in cosmetic products. It is estimated that about 85% of cosmetics have some form of parabens in them. They are commonly found in deodorants, lotions, shampoos, conditioners. Parabens mimic estrogen and contribute to the growth of breast tumor cells (MCF-7 cells). (Source: breastcancerfund.org)

Be on the lookout for any ingredient with the word "paraben" in it. There are about seven different forms of parabens, and most of them have negative impact on your body chemistry.

Fluoride

I know, I know, we've all heard that fluoride is not only safe, but that we need to supplement so we can have healthier teeth, right? That's why it's in most public water supplies and in many toothpastes. In fact, it's hard to find a toothpaste that doesn't have fluoride in it. But it can be done. So, what's all the hoopla surrounding fluoride?

At fluoride.mercola.com you can find articles about the negative aspects of fluoride. (Personally, I'm not a big fan of Dr. Mercola in general. I find him too alarmist for my preference. But, in this instance, he does share some compelling information for the case against public water fluoridation.) Fluoride, like MSG, has been called an *excitotoxin* meaning it has toxic effect on the neurological system and there are studies that suggest this may be true. Let's go back to high school Chemistry class for a few minutes to see why I'm giving fluoride a bad rap.

On a periodic table, you will notice that fluorine and its sister halogens chlorine and bromine are located just above the element Iodine. This means that in the human body, the element that is listed closest to the top of the chart, in this case fluorine and the other halogens will be absorbed before iodine. In other words, the presence of fluorine, chlorine, and bromine block the absorption of iodine.

Iodine is the primary nutrient to support the thyroid gland. How many people do you know who are on prescription medication, for life, to support their thyroid? How many of you drink from public water sources? (Are you having an "ah ha" moment, yet?) How many have had hysterectomies? How many have been diagnosed with anxiety, depression, or other neurological disorder? Do you see a possible connection? There is one. It's undeniable in my opinion, and in the opinions of those referenced on the Mercola website, and elsewhere on the web if you spend a little time looking around.

So, why not take a simple step and filter your water? You can use a filter for your drinking water. And check out the details on what all your fridge water filter addresses. Consider using toothpaste that doesn't contain fluoride. Oh, and I can't move along from this subject without touching on why this toothpaste thing is a big deal.

You may not have spent much time thinking about this before, but be sure to notice tonight when you are brushing your teeth before bed, where does the saliva with toothpaste rest in your mouth between the time you brush your teeth and you spit it out? Under your tongue. And where is one of the most direct-access-to-your-bloodstream sites in your body? Under your tongue. (That's why we use the sublingual site for application of homeopathics, silver solutions, liquid B-vitamins, and anything else we want into the bloodstream as quickly as possible.) So even though the toothpaste is somewhat diluted by your saliva, it still sits under your tongue for at least a few seconds while you brush. Most of us try to brush for as long as possible, usually 30-45 seconds or even two minutes. Thirty seconds is all your body needs to begin absorbing substances that are under the tongue. Bingo! The fluoride gets in. And boom! The iodine can't land on your cells' receptor sites. Over time, this could create a health issue. It's another avoidable health issue. Consider finding a toothpaste that doesn't contain fluoride.

Chlorine

The next big toxin we will tackle is chlorine, listed just under fluorine on the periodic table. If fluorine is in place, chlorine won't be taken in as much. Let's think about where we are getting chlorine on a daily basis. Want to guess? Even if you are filtering your drinking water, there is another place where you spend time every day and you are barraged by chlorine the entire time you are there. Swimming pool? Great guess, but every day? (Me neither.) Hot tub? Another great guess. How about your shower or bath?

Keep in mind that chlorine is a gas. We inhale it the entire time we are in the shower (unless you have a filter or are on well water). Our lungs actually have the surface space of a tennis court, so we can take in a good size amount of chlorine in a very short period of time! Chlorine is a known irritant for all respiratory issues. If someone with a known respiratory issue takes a long shower in chlorine-treated water, they are poised for a day of increased irritation. Imagine the cumulative effect over time for this person.

Filters for shower heads are easy to find at your local home store or online. They are relatively inexpensive, easy to install, and you might be surprised by the differences you notice the first week after getting the chlorine out of your shower, or bath.

If you take chlorine out of your shower, consider getting the bleach out of your home, too. I hope I haven't gone to meddlin', but bleach is the most potent form of chlorine that most people have in their homes. Those who are very concerned about the presence of any germs in their homes probably use more bleach than others. If you are concerned about how to deep clean and kill germs effectively without bleach, I can assure you it's almost fun to discover creative ways to do just this.

Some people like to make their own cleaners with essential oils and other natural cleaners.

I have to say, I'm not that person. I do have the most fabulous essential oil recipes for glass/mirror cleaner, deodorant, face wash, face serum, and face cream, but our family shops with an eco-friendly company each month and that is the primary source for our toothpaste, gum, mints, laundry detergent, other laundry additives, dishwasher detergent, dish soap, hand soap, stain remover, air freshener, toilet bowl cleaner, general cleaner, furniture polish - you get the idea. It's very economical, environmentally responsible, non-toxic, and even fun! Before we switched from toxic household cleaners to non-toxic, I had bronchitis at least twice a year and sometimes three or four times in a winter. Once we got those harmful chemicals out of our home, there was a dramatic improvement in my health.

Aluminum

Aluminum has been implicated in neurological issues, especially Alzheimer's. Around the house, it's most commonly found in cookware because it is an effective conductor of heat. Most cookware these days does not have aluminum on the outside of it, but most if not all non-stick cookware contains aluminum as a heat conductor in one of its base layers. So, if you accidentally forget to use a plastic utensil to flip that bacon, and you accidentally scratch the nonstick surface of that nonstick cookware, you may be exposing yourself and your family to aluminum. Aluminum is leached into the foods you cook and absorbed into the bloodstream. Sadly, the molecules in aluminum are small enough to cross the blood-brain barrier and over time it is suspected to accumulate in brain tissue leading to dementia or even Alzheimer's. If you have old scratched up nonstick cookware in your kitchen, don't even donate it, just toss it out. Stainless steel, glass or cast-iron cookware are aluminum-free options I can recommend.

Like aluminum foil, another more obvious culprit for aluminum is the aluminum cans that contain soft drinks and other beverages. That is the same kind of aluminum we just talked about and yes, it can and will end up in your bloodstream.

Maybe the least obvious culprit for aluminum in your home is in antiperspirant. Antiperspirants pack a double whammy, especially for women. I want to stretch you to consider exploring a different option for this one as much as possible and here's why.

Antiperspirants contain aluminum which is easily absorbed into the skin and then into the bloodstream. That alone is probably a good enough reason to avoid them altogether. But in the female body, the stakes get even higher. Let's review a little bit of anatomy. Just beneath the skin we have lymphatic channels throughout our bodies. These lymphatic channels serve as "trash cans" of sorts to collect "trash" from our bloodstream. We get into the lymph system more thoroughly in chapter four, but this is so important I want to go ahead and touch on it right here. These lymphatic channels run from below our ears, down the neck and *chest into the arms* and down into the abdominal region on both sides, then down into the legs.

The lymphatic channels go from the chest into the arms, (and there is a *lot* of lymphatic tissue in the breast area). The armpit is an important intersection of lymph and circulatory channels. In fact, at the armpit, the lymph nodes are able to release some toxins via extra sweat glands in the area. This is an important channel of elimination for the thoracic (ribs/chest) area. But what if we block this essential elimination by preventing sweat from the armpit area by using antiperspirant? Over time, it is suspected that toxins will continue to accumulate in the lymph nodes. If the body is not able to eliminate them, they can develop irregular cells and disease can set up camp. It could develop in the lymphatic tissues themselves, or in the nearby breast tissue. Are you following me?

In my opinion, this is an unnecessary risk. Everyone sweats. Yes, nervous sweat may smell a bit more than exercise sweat, and it can be a bit embarrassing to raise our arms during an important talk to reveal our nervousness to the entire room, but we have to make a choice. Will we let the rest of the world discover that we are as human as they are, or will choose to block important detoxification systems in our own bodies and risk developing an avoidable disease?

When I learned about all this, I felt convicted and challenged to stop using antiperspirant on a daily basis. I discovered effective aluminum-free deodorants that take care of the smell, and even though I still sweat, I haven't had that "Oh my gosh, look at her wet armpits!" moment during an important talk.

I've also discovered that when my eating is mostly clean and I'm not eating junk food, I have very little if any body odor at all.

Keep in mind that with aluminum, chlorine, fluorine, and parabens, occasional use/exposure is unavoidable. We don't know what kinds of skillets our food from a restaurant is cooked in. Most of us aren't going to carry a shower filter to every hotel when we are away from home, we don't and can't know every single exposure. And that's okay. There's no need to fret about those unavoidable toxin exposures. Plus, our bodies are made to detox! They can sustain a pretty heavy toxic load for a long time. I feel like we are being better stewards of our bodies when we avoid the toxic exposures we can. I can't imagine how you could to try avoid every possible exposure.

While many of the chemicals that make the air inside of our home more toxic than the air outside are from household cleaners, there may also be off-gassing from carpet, floor sealers, paint, cabinet surfaces - you get the idea. No, we aren't going to pull up all the carpet, tear out the walls, and live in a pristine unbleached canvas tent. But we can reduce the toxic load in our home by choosing non-toxic cleaners and other products when possible.

The crazy thing about toxic chemicals in the list of products above is that they don't wash off, wash out, or dry off. They linger. They leave an almost invisible residue on your clothes, dishes, and household surfaces. That residue may release chemicals into the air in your home. Did you know the EPA (Environmental Protection Agency) has said that the air INSIDE your home is up to 95% MORE TOXIC than the air OUTSIDE? Is that surprising to you? It was a shock to me the first time I heard it!

It is important for us to be aware of the presence of physical toxins so we can reduce them and help our body eliminate them. In chapter five, we will begin identifying and addressing emotional toxins. We know that both physical *and* emotional toxins affect our bodies, but do you realize your body responds to them the same exact way? You read that right. Your body doesn't know the difference between physical or emotional stress. It has one stress reaction, and that response usually involves inflammation. When we think of inflammation, we think of redness, pain, and swelling. You may be wondering if your emotions really create a reaction like that in your body. Yes, they really do.

Chapter Three

Your Body is a Temple - Keep it Clean

Your body is an amazing creation. The hypothalamus in your brain is constantly monitoring various levels in your body, everything from blood pressure to hormones to enzymes, toxins, and beyond. Then with quicker-than-lightning speed, it can dispatch appropriate responses to ensure these important levels stay within healthy ranges. It works day and night to ensure balance throughout your body.

Meanwhile, your incredible immune system is on vigilant guard for any foreign invaders (viruses, bacteria, and parasites). It has a memory even better than an elephant's, and it never forgets a single invader from the past and it is always ready to engage "troops" to fight the old or new invaders.

These are just two quick examples of the intricate feedback loops that are constantly working on behalf of your body and your overall health. I could go on and on talking about more examples, but since this is not an anatomy and physiology class, and you may not share my enthusiasm for these tiny details in your body, let's move on! Although the more I have learned about the "bazillions" of microscopic details that are in and constantly taking place in our bodies, the bigger God seems to me. He constantly reveals Himself in His creation. I am in awe!

Let's get back to some simple, but powerful habits we can develop to better steward this complex temple that is ours for life. Your body is designed to detoxify itself. You may even recognize a place or two that could benefit from some additional support.

Six Channels of Elimination

There are six main channels for elimination in our body. Each of these serves the essential task of eliminating toxins, wastes, and even excesses that our body either can't use or doesn't need at this time. As you can imagine, as long as each of them is working at the top of its game, life is pretty hunky dory. Things are going well with us! But, if one of them is overly challenged, the others will work extra hard to make up for it. That is usually fine, but if two or more are struggling, we may begin to notice a decline in our overall health.

These six channels of elimination for toxins in our bodies are lungs, kidneys, liver, lymph, colon, and skin. Okay, if you want to get technical, since we have two lungs and two kidneys, there are actually eight organs involved, but think of them as six channels for eliminating waste and toxins.

Have you ever known someone who has issues or eruptions on their skin? How do they usually treat that? Topically? Sure they do. If they develop a rash or hives, they usually apply some kind of ointment to soothe the skin. And that's fine for temporary relief of a topical symptom. But, do you ever wonder *why* the rash or eruption started in the first place? I wonder about those kinds of things. I'm naturally curious and want to understand the WHY beyond every symptom. And in this example of skin issues, I usually find that one or more of the other channels of elimination may be stressed.

The good news is that there are some relatively simple and even inexpensive steps we can take to help to help keep our organs of elimination working efficiently. While this is not a comprehensive list, it is one that I believe will help you support your body during this season of releasing emotional pain, (beginning in chapter five) which actually results in the release of physical toxins into your bloodstream. I want you to feel healthy, energetic, and strong during this healing process.

Three Simple Steps for Detoxifying Your Body

Let's explore three simple steps for supporting our body during a time of detoxification. While we could focus on any of the elimination channels, let's keep our focus on the lymphatic system for now.

Keep in mind, as you get into the later chapters, the emotional release you will experience as a result of extending forgiveness to others WILL trigger a REAL and physical release in your body. While you would be able to progress through your forgiveness list without taking the following steps, I believe these three activities will augment your body's elimination processes as you forgive. This is probably a new concept for you to take in. You may not have thought about the effect emotions have on your physical body. It is a real deal!

Ancient Chinese Secrets

In Chinese medicine (which has been practiced and documented for over 2500 years, compared to Western medicine's 150 years . . . I believe we can learn from older forms of medicine, don't you?) we learn that there are specific emotions related to specific organs. Below is a list of a few of these associations.

Organ	Emotion
Liver/Gallbladder	Anger
Heart	Anger and Shock
Lungs	Grief
Stomach	Disgust
Kidneys/Knees	Fear
Pancreas/	Joy

Consider some of these common sayings, "That makes me sick to my stomach." We usually say that when we are disgusted, don't we? Do you see the connection between the stomach and disgust?

Or, "I was so scared I almost peed my pants!" And, "His knees were knocking from fear of what would happen next!" Traditional Chinese Medicine recognizes a connection between the kidneys, the knees, and the emotion of fear.

Or, "She really has a lot of gall to do that!" What feeling are we usually having when we say that? We are usually angry. The gallbladder is an important little pouch near the liver. The liver is related to anger. Don't you find these possible connections interesting?

It just makes sense to support these organs of elimination as we release emotions (and even toxins) through the process of giving forgiveness. Three simple steps to physically support this detoxification process are:

- **Breathe**

- **Bathe**

- **Brush**

The first technique is something you are already doing . . . so we are just going to tweak it a bit for some different results!

Breathe

There's no doubt that you are already breathing. If you weren't, well, I don't believe you would have made it this far into the book! But there's a difference between our regular involuntary breathing and deep breathing.

Deep breathing blesses our bodies in many ways. It increases oxygen in our bloodstream and in our cells. It massages the internal organs in our abdomen, and it stimulates lymphatic flow (which stimulates our immune system). It only takes a few minutes to do, and we usually feel relaxed, refreshed and rested afterward.

It isn't difficult to do, but there is a bit of technique to doing it properly. Begin by lying down on your back. Place a pillow on top of your abdomen. Now, take a deep breath in. Did the pillow move? No? Then, let's try it again, this time with the intention of moving that abdomen and the pillow toward the ceiling as you inhale, then lowering them as you exhale.

Have you ever watched a baby sleeping? When my daughter Bailey was a newborn, I could get lost for literal hours just watching her sleep! And one thing I noticed was that her little bottom and tummy rose and fell with each breath. She didn't seem to breathe from her chest and shoulders as most adults do . . . but she was breathing the way God made her to breathe, and she was breathing deeply.

Years later I would learn that indeed, that rising and falling tummy was the key to deep, cleansing breathing. But, if you ask most people to take a deep breath, you will see their shoulders go up toward their ears, then fall back down. As it turns out, our diaphragm muscle which is located in our upper abdomen under our lungs is responsible for the expansion and contraction of our lungs. So, when we take a really good, deep, cleansing breath, our abdomen/tummy will go away from our core, then return.

Okay American women, I know this goes against everything we know about holding our tummies in at all times! We would just rather …well, we would rather not let our tummies out for anything! So may I just give you permission once and for all, in the interest of the great health God designed you to enjoy, to let that tummy out girl and breathe! If this is just more than you are ready to do in public, it's okay to start out as a "closet breather" and practice only in the privacy of your own home.

But I do hope you will take a few minutes every day, maybe upon awakening and again before drifting off to sleep for the night, to breathe in deeply through your nose. Hold it for about 15 seconds, then slowly exhale through your mouth as your count to 20. Breathing deeply and slowly will not result in hyperventilation. Take your time. Bless your body. There are even apps for your smartphone that will chime every 15 minutes throughout the day to remind you to take that deep breath. I once shared an office with a chiropractor who had that app. Hearing its "gong" sound helped both of us remember during our busy days to stop and breathe. Yea, being reminded to breathe deeply is that important!

Bathe

The second temple cleaning technique you are probably already doing at least sometimes, **Bathe**! Okay, I get it, some people just are not bath-takers. There are shower people, and there are bath people. Some people bathe and others shower, but many shower people do not like to bathe. They lament, "What do I do while I am sitting in the tub?!" They don't have time to soak in a bath. They just want get in and out of the shower and be done.

Will you judge me if I confess to being a full-on shower person? Seriously, our current home doesn't even have a tub! We are all shower people around this place. But, this technique of bathing and soaking is so beneficial, we find creative ways to experience the benefits even without a tub in our home. So whether you have a fabulous jet-tub, a tub/shower combo, or only showers, you can still benefit from this kind of bathing.

The key to therapeutic bathing/soaking is Epsom salt. Your grandmother may have had you take an Epsom salt bath when you were a kid. I never liked those because they made my skin tingle, but it turns out that tingling is therapeutic! If you have a tub, run the water as warm as is comfortable, add a couple handfuls of Epsom Salt, climb in and soak for 15-20 minutes. (If you can stick it out 40 minutes, you will get double advantages.) While you are soaking, your body is absorbing the magnesium and other nutrients from the salt in the water. You will feel relaxed, but it also facilitates your body's ability to cleanse and detox.

*Note: **If your blood pressure tends to run on the lower side**, may I suggest that instead of Epsom Salts, you use Baking Soda and salt? The Magnesium in Epsom Salts has been known to help lower blood pressure. If your blood pressure is already on the low side, an Epsom Salt bath or soak may not be a good experience for you.*

If you don't have a tub, you can get a similar benefit from creating a Foot Soak. Find a tub big enough to place your feet in (dish tubs from retailers work great for most feet) place one handful of Epsom Salt (or Baking Soda) into the tub, add water as warm as you can tolerate, and soak your feet for 15 – 20 minutes. If you're a rush-rush shower-taker and you aren't sure what to do while your feet soak, this is a great time to catch up on reading that book that has been gathering dust on your nightstand, or just sit there and practice deep breathing. You may also wish to add essential oils to your bath or soak. Lavender essential oil is known to be soothing and relaxing. Orange, Lemon, or Bergamot essential oils are more stimulating. I don't recommend peppermint or other strong oils in a bath, because it can cause a burning sensation in sensitive areas! But they are usually fine in a foot soak.

If you want to make it a family affair, grab a tub for each family member, gather round and soak, laugh at yourselves, make funny memories of soaking your feet together, and just enjoy your time together. (A practical tip here, be sure to have a towel ready to catch your dripping feet once the soaking time is over. Otherwise, you may feel grumbly tracking your wet toes through the house to the towels!) There is no need to rinse your feet after soaking, just dry them off and you are back in business. Resist the temptation to do this in front of the TV or scrolling through social media. Let this be a time when you are either quiet, connecting with others, or laughing. Let it be a time of relaxation in the present moment. Afterward, your body will feel relaxed, so enjoy.

Perhaps you are wondering how often you should bathe or soak. Once a week is an excellent start, but if you feel like doing it more often, go for it!

Brush

The third temple cleaning technique is **brush** (your skin, that is!) Have you heard of skin brushing? I hadn't either until I attended a class on natural health several years ago. The presenter was absolutely enthralled with this method of supporting the body's detoxification pathways of lymph, skin, and boosting circulation. She made it sound like the best thing in the whole world! I began to ask myself, how could I have lived 40 years without experiencing the many benefits of this eighth wonder?

As you might imagine, I went out with great excitement and anticipation and bought a skin brush, then proceeded to brush my whole body just as instructed. But, instead of awakening the next day to feelings of renewed energy, zeal, and near super hero status, I felt terrible. What?! This utter malaise was not what the speaker had described at all. How was this even possible? I was disappointed and just generally bummed, plus I felt sick. No fun at all! Do you have any idea why it all happened that way? Did I do something wrong? Did I buy the wrong brush?

Skin brushing is unbelievably simple. It only takes a few minutes to do a thorough job, once you get the hang of it. But, it's pretty powerful! Let me explain a bit about the lymphatic system.

You know how your street looks the day that everyone sets out their trash for the waste management folks? All those cans are set out in a line until the truck comes along and empties them. If they sit there long enough, they get stinky from all the garbage inside. If they never got moved, their contents would putrify, gross things would begin to grow inside them, and well, you can easily imagine the grossness that would ensue. Let's move on.

Inside your body is a network of lymph nodes, not too dissimilar from trash cans. They exist to catch waste from blood cells who are scavenging the blood stream for various kinds of "trash". They may contain dead blood cells, viruses, bacteria, parasites, and even toxins from our diet and environment. An interesting thing about these lymph nodes is that they don't have a trash truck to come empty them from time to time. They don't even have a pump to regularly remove their contents. The primary strategy for them to release their contents so they can be removed from your body is this . . . **you must move your body**. That's right. Your lymph system doesn't have a pump of its own. By contrast, the circulatory system has the heart to pump blood, and the respiratory system has the lungs to pump oxygen into the cells. But if you don't move your body, the lymph nodes will simply continue to collect waste from your body. Over time, they may swell, you may develop infection, your body temperature may rise and you may become ill.

But, when you move your body on a regular basis, as we will discuss more in the next chapter, your lymph system is better equipped to perform its job more efficiently. So, what does this have to do with my feeling terrible after I brushed my skin for the first time? At that time in my life, I did not yet see or practice the benefits of exercising on a daily basis. I would take an *occasional* walk, bike ride, hike, or even jog, but I didn't have a plan to move my body in an aerobic way on a regular basis. So, my lymph nodes were likely full of "garbage" and beyond ready for the trash man to come clean them out.

When I skin brushed for the first time, it stimulated circulation and release of toxins from my congested lymph nodes. When those toxins hit my blood stream, my other organs of elimination were overwhelmed and I felt terrible from having so much junk floating around in my bloodstream. As you can imagine, I didn't become an advocate for this practice after the first time, or the second time, or even the third or fourth time. In fact, every time I Skin Brushed, I felt really badly the next day! You may be wondering why I would even suggest that you skin brush after reading my own experience, but stay with me.

Then I realized, and this is really important, I *need* to support this important system of my body. Maybe I didn't have to do my whole body every time. So, I decided to take a gentler approach, literally brushing just one limb (one arm or one leg) a day, sometimes every other day. With this gentler approach, I knew I was experiencing benefits, but I didn't feel as bad. I even noticed I had improved sensory/ touch perception on my arms after brushing them. I could actually feel temperature in the air for the first time in a long time. That was a big deal for me! Plus, my entire circulatory system thanked me, too! I noticed my hands and feet weren't as cold as they used to be.

While it's been said that our skin renews itself every seven years, I am now an enthusiastic advocate for brushing it regularly to keep the extra dead skin cells off, to stimulate the lymph flow through the lymph nodes located just beneath the skin, and to boost overall circulation. Some have even reported a decrease in cellulite after a few months of faithful skin brushing. While I make no promises about that one, I can say I have experienced it myself and have known others who have enjoyed this benefit as well!

How to Skin Brush

Now that you know you may need to start slowly, are you eager to experience this health-empowering practice for yourself? The first thing you need is a skin brush. These are usually sold in the bath and shower accessory section of the store. The most important feature to look for in a skin brush is natural fibers. Typically, there is a long, removable wooden handle, and an oval brush with light-colored natural fibers.

You can skin brush either before or after a shower or bath. There are different schools of thought on whether it's better to brush before or after a bath or shower, but I find them both inconclusive to my own satisfaction. Brush when it works best for you. Your preference is the better option for you. If you brush afterward, be sure your skin is completely dry before brushing.

You will begin at either your foot or your hand. In small, short, light strokes, you will brush toward your heart. This does not mean one, long stroke from fingertip to heart. There are many, short brush strokes up the arm or leg, slowly moving toward the general direction of the heart.

The strokes are similar to strokes you make when brushing off lint from a garment. Just a quick flick of the wrist gets the job done.

Repeat up both legs, both arms, and on your trunk and torso, always brushing toward the heart.

Why brush toward the heart? It is the biggest pump in your body. It's already pumping so you are stimulating circulation toward the pump. Don't overthink this. Just brush. And notice how invigorated your skin feels afterward. You may even notice a boost in your energy throughout the day.

What if you feel terrible after a skin brushing? I hope this doesn't happen to you, but if it does, please don't give up on this valuable practice. Just slow down a bit, consider brushing just one limb each day, or every other day. Be sure you are drinking plenty of water and consider adding a walk to your day to further boost lymphatic activity. Persist, and know that you are blessing your body as you release toxic emotions, and physical toxins, too!

So, which of the three techniques for detoxing will you try first? Deep breathing? Bathing? Or skin brushing? You may want to begin with one for a week, then try another for a week, then try the third for a week . . . or you may want to jump into all three with great gusto! Whichever approach you choose will bless your body. And if you notice a headache, body aches, or other malaise, just slow down, drink extra water, move your body more, and don't give up.

Chapter Four

Walking is Good for Your Soul

The fact you are reading this book right now suggests you are a person committed to lifelong learning. That being said, it's highly likely that you've already heard about the cardiovascular benefits of regular exercise. You probably know that it increases the strength of the heart muscle, the lungs, and it releases endorphins (feel-good hormones) into your bloodstream.

Prior to reading this book, you may or may not have known that your lymphatic system doesn't have a pump of its own, so in order for it to release the toxins collected in the body-wide lymph glands, it requires movement. We touched on this in the last chapter as it related to detoxifying your body. Walking, running, and jumping on a trampoline (large or small) are all excellent methods of stimulating the lymphatic system. With every step, every motion of your body moving up then down, the lymph glands are " pumped" to help you get rid of toxins that we all accumulate in everyday life, no matter how "clean" we try to live.

I believe walking is a great form of physical activity for every body. If you are a runner, keep up the great work! I'm so happy you love running! We all rejoice with you and are even inspired by you, but if you're not a runner, I still love ya!

When I was in my early forties, I accepted a challenge (from a book I was reading) to begin to walk five days a week, at least 30 minutes, no matter what! The author promised all kinds of perks from this seemingly simple daily activity. At that point, I was pretty much desperate for some physical breakthroughs, so I didn't just give it a whirl, I committed, and I did it! And for the most part, I still do it several years later.

Since we lived on a busy highway at that time, and I didn't really want to walk 30 minutes a day in our horse arena, I had to find a place nearby to walk. The closest places were about a 15-minute drive, so I initially settled on walking around a pretty little lake in Bella Vista, Arkansas. It was a nice two-mile walk and some days I would extend my distance. I committed to walk at least five days a week, unless the temperatures were below 34 degrees (that is just my personal tolerance threshold) or if it was raining pretty hard. Wouldn't you know, we had one of the mildest winters on record that year! I hardly missed a single day for the first three and a half years. When we traveled, we would find places to walk. Unless I was running a fever or the roads were impassable due to snow or ice, I walked.

What had started as a quest for some physical breakthrough quickly began to yield some of those "perks" I had read about, but so many more that I hadn't expected. Sometimes when the weather wasn't cooperating, I would pop in a DVD and do a workout inside. But you know, that didn't offer the same experience. Yes, my heart rate would increase, I would sweat, push myself just enough to be good and sore for a few days afterward, but I longed for "my" walk.

"My" walk became a sacred time, usually to myself. Sometimes I would invite Tim or Bailey to come along, but most of the time it was just me. It eventually became an invitation-only event in which my family assumed I would go solo, unless I invited them to come along. But I wasn't alone. Sure, there were other walkers out there, but even when none of them was in sight, I knew I wasn't alone. My walk time became a designated time most mornings when I would hush, be silent, and listen to my Father. It was astonishing that He had so much to say to me that I just hadn't been able to hear in the hustle and bustle of my daily life.

I remember one particular walk, this time in a city park, when I was the only one out there. That day I had a bone to pick with the Father. I was literally walking, throwing my hands up in the air, and raising my voice to Him. He was reminding me about a special assignment He had given me, and I was reminding Him that I had heard His yoke is easy and His burden is light (Matthew 11:30), but it just didn't feel like that to me! I needed Him to pull off some pretty specific details in order for me to be able to do what He asked me to do. It was way beyond what I could do on my own, but I reminded Him that if it was important to Him, it was important to me, but I needed his help.

Don't you wish you could have watched this walk from one of the nearby houses? It had to be humorous – and puzzling - to the observer! WHY was this grown woman screaming and throwing her arms about when there was no one else around? What was she saying? To whom did she think she was speaking? Oh, if they only knew! And do you know what happened next?

My eyes fell upon something that literally directed my path to first one person, then another, and by the end of that very day, God Himself had filled in ALL the details . . . no more excuses . . . and I launched the very first ever Healthy Body study group less than two weeks later. He provided a location, the participants, and a host of other details. It was stunning! And I believe it wouldn't have happened that way if I had not set aside time in my schedule to walk daily, to listen, to talk, and to watch Him move. As you read the next few pages about the benefits of moving your body, please don't limit your expectations of what the benefits are to what you read on these pages. Open your sense of exploration and expectation for encountering the Father on a daily basis, in a new way. Yes, I usually have my daily quiet time of Bible study after my walk, while I finish sweating, but this walking thing really took me to a whole new level in relationship with Him. It is my prayer that you will encounter Him freshly as well.

When we walk at a brisk enough pace to require pacing our breathing (as if you are going somewhere and you need to get there as quickly as possible), every inhale results in essential oxygen being literally pushed into our cells, and every exhale takes with it carbon dioxide and a host of other toxic chemicals from the cells in our body. It is really quite an impressive exchange that takes place with every single breath. Especially when we are "winded".

You know how you can "see your breath" on a cold day? Isn't it so very fascinating to actually be able to SEE your breath? Of course, what we are seeing are frozen particles of water that are being expelled from our body. But within those tiny water droplets, toxic poisons are being released. We probably don't really think too much about this process most of the time. After all, it is just one of those things that has a way of happening. I think it's super cool that even though we don't SEE our breath in all temperatures, our body is still doing what it does, helping us get rid of the bad stuff that could really trip us up in our physical health department if we leave it inside us. Can you see how something as simple as walking could really be a literal first step to turning your health around? Isn't this exciting!

I'm focusing on walking because it is relatively low impact, free or cheap for anyone to do, and pretty much safe for anyone who is able to walk at all. But if your love is running, fitness classes, fitness DVDs, your elliptical, or anything else, that's fine, too. While you will gain cardiovascular benefits from all the above, it just doesn't offer the same quiet, reflective time that I have found in walking.

When you walk outside, you have the opportunity to experience even more of God's glory through His creation. Now, be sure you hear me here, I did not say that we want to glorify creation. We know that He *reveals His nature* through creation. In the King James Version, Psalm 19:1 says, "The heavens declare the glory of God; and the firmament (vast expanse of the sky) shows His handiwork." We honor the Creator, not the creation. Do you see the difference here?

And oh how His creation demonstrates His creativity! No two sunsets are ever the same, nor are two sunrises. Each day I walk down our dirt road where we live now, I notice subtle differences from the day before. Maybe it's a stalk of wild sunflowers that's just about to burst into bloom, or maybe its season for bloom has ended with the first frost. Maybe it's the way the sun illuminates the water droplets on the spider webs that appeared overnight. Or, on a wintry day, I may have the opportunity to watch bald eagles soaring overhead. There are so many tiny details you notice at the pace of a walk that you might miss at a run, or on a bike, and certainly if zooming by in a car. Slow down or stop and take in the wonder.

All creation reveals the glory of its Creator. If you've ever wondered if God is interested in the details of your life, may I invite you to find a dirt road to walk down? Observe the countless details He has put into place. The tiny petals on wildflowers. The buzzing of a bumble bee as he pollinates. The provision of water made for wildlife through natural drainage. Even the breath of fresh air. Details are important to God. You are important to God. And I believe there are some things in His creation He has put there at just the right time for our enjoyment. Savor this gift in your day. He's lovin' on ya!

Obviously, I get tremendous enjoyment from my walks down our little country road. But before we moved to our current home, I found other places of beauty to walk. It has been a lovely trend that so many communities are creating green spaces and walking/biking trails for us to enjoy. I'm pretty sure that wherever you live, there is a beautiful space nearby just waiting for you to discover it and its many tiny wonders.

Is walking the best exercise? I don't know. Is it a complete exercise? Not really. I find that supplementing a walking program with some sort of upper body resistance training lends itself to a more balanced program. Weights, resistance bands, or even exercises using your own body weight as resistance are all great options.

But as I said earlier, walking is easily accessible, relatively cheap and it's super easy to share! Do invest in a good pair of shoes, and get new ones about every 6 months. I'm often asked by clients, "Which exercise is the best for me?" My favorite responses to that question are:

1. Find something you love to do that you WILL do; and

2. Find someone you love to do it WITH.

You don't have to have someone to walk with, but especially in the beginning it may be helpful for accountability purposes to know that someone else is waiting for you to walk each day. Don't wait until you have someone to go with you, though. Be sure you are in a safe area, then get out there and get started.

"When is the best time to exercise?" This is another question that can trip some people up. For me, it is usually first thing in the morning. If it doesn't happen then, there is a 90% chance it won't happen at all that day, no matter how good my intentions, or even how firm my plans are. But I know many committed walkers who have set aside time to get out there after work, or after school, or after the kids' nap, or after whatever else happens during your day. Find a time that you can commit to, and start there. If you need to change the time of day you walk at some point, that's okay, too.

My purpose in encouraging you to begin a walking/physical activity program is NOT to create another program or rule in your life. The purpose here to open a door to increased peace, strength, health, confidence, hope, wonder, and the list could go on and on. Why not commit this week to walk five times? If you haven't been physically active in a while, start with 10 minutes of walking each day. That is a great start! Then, as you feel yourself getting stronger (and you will condition more quickly than you expect!) add five more minutes, then five more, and so on. If you are already doing some other kind of fitness activity, may I invite you to give a simple walk a try? You might discover something you had no idea you had been missing!

As we wrap up our time on "the walk", let me clarify that the walking I'm talking about, thirty minutes a day at a fairly rapid clip, probably won't lead to massive weight loss. Please don't confuse this kind of walking with a miraculous weight loss cure. Recently on a morning walk, one of my neighbors drove by and we visited for a bit.

He commented on my walking habits. Out of my mouth blurted, "It may not make me skinny, but it sure does make me happy!" That pretty much sums it up.

This kind of walking is primarily for our mental and emotional health. While yes, there will be physical perks that we've already covered, maybe even some weight loss, I want to be sure you don't have unrealistic expectations about the benefits of a peaceful walking program. Most people will need to have a more aggressive kind of exercise program if its primary purpose is weight loss. That's okay, too. In fact, that's really great! I'm not going to get into the benefits, the how-to's, your why, or program specifics here, but I will encourage you to get out there and commit to "the walk". It will bless you in ways you probably can't imagine, until you experience it.

Chapter Five

Forgiveness is a Gift You Give Yourself

We've spent the first few chapters of this book laying a firm foundation for your physical health. By now, you've likely discovered the powerful connection between your mood and food, the value of intentional nutrition in your life, the surprising presence of toxins all around you and everywhere you go, the power of water in your body, and maybe even some other new discoveries you hadn't heard of before reading Healthy Body. Now it's time for you to begin to experience the super power of forgiveness in a fresh way that will forever improve your life and your relationships.

But did you know that your spirit and emotions are intricately woven into and throughout your physical body? Every emotional experience affects you physically, every physical experience affects you emotionally, every spiritual experience affects you physically and emotionally, just as every food and drink choice you make affects your mind, body and spirit. So, as you continue to make healthier food and drink choices, let's take some time to address the hurts from your past that may unknowingly be affecting your physical and emotional health.

When we hold onto hurts and negative emotions, it creates measurable stress on our physical bodies. And as we learned, the body doesn't know the difference between emotional stress and physical stress. When we hold on to past hurts, or when they still bother us emotionally, the body responds in the same way it does when we eat junk food or don't drink enough water: toxic stress builds up in the body, reducing our ability to heal and creating a measurable, negative effect on our physical health. Forgiveness is the antidote to this toxic build-up of emotions.

Let's take a few minutes to seek the Word about the power of forgiveness. In Matthew 6:14 (New International Version) we read, "For if you forgive men when they sin against you, your heavenly Father will also forgive you. But, if you do not forgive men their sins, your Father will not forgive your sins." Let me point out that these words were spoken by Jesus. And this is big stuff! IF we forgive men, our Father will forgive us. Conversely, if we don't forgive men, our Father will not forgive us. Can you see that this must be a very important principle for Jesus to speak of it? We all need the forgiveness of our Father for the wrong things we have done in our lives.

Before we move along, I would like to take just a moment to be very clear about something related to forgiveness. As you begin to think about the people who have hurt you in the past, you likely are feeling hurt from the pain of past events. I want to acknowledge the fact that the people who have hurt you may have done something very terrible to you. They may have hurt you in ways that have had long-term effects. They may have hurt someone you love dearly. *You may think they do not **deserve** forgiveness.* So let me ask you this, do you deserve the forgiveness you have so generously received from our Father? I don't, either. So, let's apply some grace (unmerited favor or something good we don't deserve) to this situation, and choose to forgive, in spite of the wrong actions of others. You will come to see that ***forgiveness is not a feeling, it is a decision***.

Forgiving someone does **not** make what they did right. Forgiving them does not mean you are reconciled in a relationship. Forgiving them does **not** mean you will spend the holidays together. Forgiveness *may not do a thing for them*. But it does a lot for you! When you forgive, your Father will forgive you. When you forgive, you are brought into a restored relationship with the Father. He loves that! You love that!

Besides, who are we to *judge* whether something is forgivable or not? In Matthew 7:1-2 (NIV) we read, "Do not judge, or you too will be judged. For in the same way you judge others, you will be judged, and with the same measure you use, it will be measured to you."

When it comes to being judged, I don't want justice, I want mercy! I don't want to judge others at all. I don't want to be judged by others, either. My prayer is, "Lord, help me to not judge others, not here, not on the road, not at the mall, not at work, not in my family. Show me ways I have judged others, and forgive me for each one of them."

Let us not judge others. Let's choose to forgive them. "Father forgive them . . ." These were some of Jesus' final words. This suggests these words are very important. He measured their value, and spoke of forgiveness. It's important. It's essential. Let's just do it! And let's do it NOW!

One of my earliest memories with the power of forgiveness took place shortly before I married. As a child, I experienced the pain of sexual abuse. In my psychology studies in college, I had come to understand there could be far-reaching effects on my marriage relationship as a result of the abuse. I was convicted of the importance of forgiving the abuser from my childhood before I entered my marriage. I didn't want to carry any of that old "junk" into my new marital relationship.

So, one night, alone in my room, I remember sitting on the side of my bed and praying to forgive the perpetrator. I felt a sense of relief and peace. I didn't feel like I needed to invite him to my wedding or have any further relationship with him, but I felt like the hurts of my past would remain there, in the past, and that I could look forward to moving on in a healthy marriage relationship.

As much as I'd like to tell you that everything was just fine from that point on, that wouldn't be the truth. But I did feel a settled peace for taking the steps toward forgiving the person who had caused me the most hurt up to that point in my life. And yet, any time I remembered the past abuse, I still felt pain. Although I thought I had forgiven my perpetrator, I continued to struggle with deep emotional pain until my early 40's. Psychology didn't quite offer all the solutions I had hoped.

If you knew me during my younger years, you may have noticed I was usually smiling. Most people who knew me then thought I had it all together. I made good grades in school. I set a good example for other kids. I was responsible and dependable at work. I was a GG (good girl) who didn't do "bad" things. So on the outside, it looked pretty good.

What you couldn't see was that inside, under those smiles, was my pain. I cried myself to sleep many nights. I was in pain from things that had happened to me. I was in pain because I couldn't forgive myself. I was in pain because I felt like no matter how hard I tried, it wasn't good enough. *I wasn't good enough.* So, I tried harder. I tried so very hard to do the right thing. I tried so hard to please other people, even when I was emotionally depleted. I tried so hard to do more, more, more. And then one day, I simply couldn't do more, anymore.

In the twelve years following college, I worked in corporate America, worked in social services, broke my back during pregnancy, became a mom, lost my dad, dealt with my mother's health issues, launched a church plant with my husband, and enjoyed success in the direct sales industry. Eventually all the stressors and unresolved conflicts caught up with me.

In my early thirties, I developed disabling vertigo and weakness. I could no longer care for my daughter, with whom I was staying home to raise and enjoy. What should have been one of the most joyful times of my life turned into months of visits to specialists and many tests. Eventually, the doctors told me it was all "in my head" and sent me home to figure out how to navigate this new life though it was hardly living at all.

Through a series of God-ordered events, I was introduced to the healing principles of natural health and nutrition and was able to quickly regain my ability to perform daily functions. I went on to complete my studies with Trinity College of Natural Health and began working with clients. Although I found my work tremendously satisfying, I couldn't help but feel there was still something missing. I also began to develop an increasing number of food sensitivities.

A few years into my practice, I began to notice that some of my clients seemed to "hit a wall" in their healing process. They would progress along to a certain point, then their progress seemed to stall. I suspected there may have been some kind of spiritual issues at play in these situations, but I didn't know how to help them.

In 2010, I attended Wellspring School of Supernatural Ministry in Anchorage, Alaska for the purpose of learning some new techniques to help my clients.

While there, I experienced the healing power of forgiveness personally and learned to address many supernatural strongholds in my life. As I learned to forgive and let go of bitterness, fear, rejection, and even self-hatred, I was healed of my food sensitivities! As I dug into other areas, I noticed that some of my self-destructive behaviors and feelings such as perfectionism, self-hatred, and being a control freak just seemed to vanish from my life. This experience was like finding the missing piece of a puzzle. Through learning about the authority I had in Christ and the giftings of the Holy Spirit, I was able to forgive past hurts and receive healing like never before.

Your experiences may be different than mine, but can you relate to an event like this where you were "justifiably" hurt? Is there a time or event in your relationship where trust was violated? Can you still recall the details? Does it hurt to think about it?

If you're ready to experience a sample of the freedom I'm talking about, I want you to think of a situation in which you have been hurt in the past. Allow yourself a few moments to recall a few of the details around the situation. Do you feel emotional pain when you begin to recall the particulars about the situation? If so, there is some healing getting ready to happen in your life RIGHT NOW!

Now let's purpose and choose to forgive this person you are thinking of. The way we are going to do this is by following along with a simple prayer. It's simple, but powerful! At the end of it, we are going to ask the Holy Spirit to show you the truth about the situation. (You've read that the truth is what sets us free, right?) At that time, I will ask you to be still and quiet, and to listen for something the Holy Spirit wants to show or tell you.

If you've never participated in this kind of interactive prayer, go ahead and be excited with expectation that something is getting ready to happen! After you read through this prayer, take about a minute to quietly listen, with your eyes closed. Pay attention for one or more of the following to come into your mind:

A picture

A word

A smell

A sound

A feeling

Or another thought or memory related to the situation you just prayed through.

Expect the Holy Spirit to minister uniquely to you. He loves you! He knows you intimately. He wants to show you something. Let's see what happens.

Read the following prayer out loud. It is important to do this aloud and not just in your mind. I believe the enemy may be able to plant thoughts into our minds, but I don't believe he can hear our thoughts. He can hear our words.

Forgiveness Prayer

Heavenly Father, I purpose and choose to forgive _____ (the person) for _____ (what they did, be specific). I release them and cancel their debt to me.

In the name of Jesus, I cancel all Satan's authority over me in this memory because it is forgiven.

Holy Spirit, heal my heart and show me the truth about this situation.

(Pause and listen here for at least one minute. Take longer if you need to.)

What happened after you prayed?

In ministry, I have come to believe that nothing happens until we pray. So, it's a good practice that when we want or need something to happen, we need to pray about it at once. And I believe that when we pray, things happen! We read in Matthew 16:19 and again in Matthew 18:18 that what is loosed on earth is loosed in heaven; and what is bound on earth is bound in heaven. When we pray, we are moving the heavens! Write down what the Holy Spirit reveals to you after your prayer. Begin a list of people you need to forgive. Repeat this process as many times as you need to.

Forgiveness is a super power tool in our arsenal because when we use it, or apply it to situations in our life, it brings healing to hurting relationships, it maintains healthy relationships, and it provides for healthy relationships in the future.

Whether these relationships are with a spouse, a child, a parent, a sibling, a co-worker, a boss, a neighbor, a friend, or even someone who is recklessly driving down the highway too fast or too near us, this dynamic tool will empower us to have stronger, healthier relationships in every facet of our lives! The amazing thing is this, as we experience improved relationships with other people, it actually allows us to enjoy closer fellowship with our Heavenly Father.

As I write this, I am praying for you. It is my prayer that the Holy Spirit will do a unique work in your life even before you finish this chapter. Get ready! Be expecting something in your life to change! Prepare yourself for a fresh touch of peace.

I hope you are feeling excited and that you are wanting more of this freedom! I'm going to suggest some homework before you move along to the next chapter.

Get a brand-new spiral notebook and begin writing out your Forgiveness List. Ask the Holy Spirit to bring to mind every single specific hurt, no matter how small or how big from your past. He will gently bring them to mind. Write down each one on a new line in your notebook.

After you have written down every single hurtful situation you can remember, repeat the Forgiveness Prayer for each and every single, specific situation. It may seem repetitive, but this simple prayer is no less powerful the sixtieth time you pray it than it was the first time you prayed it. Then, write down what the Holy Spirit shows you about each situation.

I do recommend keeping this list private. These are matters between you and your Heavenly Father. You do not have to go to each person and let them know you have forgiven them, unless you feel so impressed. We are not doing this for man, we are doing this for a reconciling to right relationship with our Father.

It's ok if you notice your list getting kind of long. When I started my list, I thought it would only take a few minutes, but as I asked the Holy Spirit to help me recall past hurts, He did and my list got long! I ended up with over 60 names/hurtful situations on that first list. It took several days, actually over a week before I felt like I had gotten through listing the majority of my hurts from the past.

I find that life provides new material every single day. I can't recall a day that I have not prayed the forgiveness prayer at least once, twice or more since I first learned these principles. These days, I forgive QUICKLY! I find that this reduces the likelihood of the enemy setting up a new stronghold in this area of my life. I don't want to relinquish any of the ground I have gained and I don't want you to, either. Stay up on your forgiving, the peace from this diligent work will surprise you.

Forgiveness is a Gift You Give Yourself

Chapter Six

You Are Wonderfully Made

"Next to Jesus, are you your own best friend?"

The first time I was asked that question (on a DVD I was watching), I literally threw the notebook I was taking notes in across the room! I think I even screamed at the TV, "NO! I'm my own worst enemy!" Do you ever feel that way?

As far back as I could remember, I had struggled with harsh feelings of self-disgust, impossible expectations for perfectionism, and being a control freak. I never liked the look of my thighs. No matter what I did, I wasn't good *enough* at anything I did, even when I received recognition from others. I was easily angered at myself for even the slightest mistake. I was constantly saying negative things to myself, and it was really like living in a pressure cooker – stuck there with myself – all the time. No Bueno!

Common phrases I would say to myself included,

"That was stupid!"

"I am such an idiot!"

"Duh! Didn't I THINK before I did that?!"

"I'll never be good enough."

"I can't ever get it right!"

May I ask you a question? Would you ever talk to anyone else the way you talk to yourself?

I'd guess you absolutely would NOT speak to anyone else the way you speak to yourself. For some reason, we buy into these lies about ourselves (which are fed to us on a continuous feed from the enemy) and we frequently condemn ourselves for not reaching impossible standards that we would never apply to anyone else, yet we quickly berate ourselves through negative self-talk. All. The. Time.

In Matthew 22:36-40 (NIV) we read about the Pharisees who were trying to trick Jesus by asking Him a nearly impossible question, "Teacher which is the great commandment in the Law?" And He said to him, "You shall love the Lord your God with all you heart, and with all your soul, and with all your mind. This is the great and foremost commandment. And a second is like it, 'You shall love your neighbor as yourself.' On these two commandments depend the whole Law and the Prophets."

Hone in on the second statement of Jesus in this passage, "You shall love your neighbor *as yourself*." If we love our neighbors as ourselves, there is an assumption that we love ourselves. Do you see that? And yet, too often, for whatever reason, we may not feel like we love ourselves. Let's talk about what some of the reasons could be for our not loving ourselves.

The first place I want to "visit" as we explore this may be one of the last places you would expect, at church. How do you see yourself in position to Father God? Do you see yourself as a loved, valuable, important son or daughter of the most High God? Or do you see yourself as a "wretch"? Have you been taught that you are lowly, worthless, scum? Or have you received revelation about how God sees you? What we hear in church penetrates our minds and our spirits. If you currently see yourself as anything less than beloved, adored, precious and valuable, may I rock your world?

In Psalm 139:14 (English Standard Version), the psalmist wrote, "I will give thanks to Thee, for I am fearfully and wonderfully made; Wonderful are Thy works, and my soul knows it very well."

We are WONDERFULLY MADE! YOU are WONDERFULLY MADE! God does not make junk. And just in case you are thinking, "Well, DiAnna, I know that He doesn't make junk, but I have done a fine job messing up His creation through my own mistakes" be comforted by the truth that He is *still making* you. He will bring good from the "mess you have made", because He is our redeemer. His being our redeemer means that He, and only He, can bring something good from something painful, ugly, and hurtful in your life. And not only can He do that, I believe He wants to do that, because He absolutely loves you!

In Psalm 139:17 (ESV) we read, "How precious also are Thy thoughts to me, O God! How vast is the sum of them!" WOW!! God's thoughts toward us are PRECIOUS (adored, cherished, dear, loved, treasured). He has placed great value on you. When He thinks of you, His thoughts are that you are adored, you are cherished, He holds you very dear to Himself. You are His beloved. He treasures you! (Does this make you feel a bit more special? Are you starting to get a clearer picture of how God sees you? I LOVE this! This is TRUTH. It's from God's Word, and I believe that right now in your heart, the Holy Spirit is confirming His truth in you.) But wait, there's more!

In Psalm 8:4-5 (New American Standard) we read "What is man that Thou dost take thought of him? And the son of man, that Thou dost care for him? Yet Thou has made him (man) a little lower than God (Jesus), and dost crown him with glory and majesty." The author goes on to marvel at how God gave man dominion over His creation.

To me, these verses do not sound like someone is talking about a "wretch". We are just a little lower than Jesus. We know we are co-heirs with Jesus. And we know that we are beloved children of an incredibly loving God. Wretch? NO! We are children of Almighty God. So I wonder, when can we start living like we know that?

Maybe church doctrine has de-railed our picture of ourselves. But maybe not.

Maybe the reason we have a lowly opinion of ourselves is that somewhere along the way, we decided we didn't like something about ourselves. Maybe it was our hair . . . or lack of. Maybe we compared ourselves to others and decided we were too fat, too skinny, too tall, or too short. Maybe our car just wasn't as cool as everyone else's.

Maybe our home wasn't as nice as the other homes in our town. Or we couldn't sing as well as the other people in church.

Maybe our parents' expectations were too much for us to live up to. Perhaps the pressure of meeting everyone else's expectations just got to us, and we started hating ourselves because we just couldn't quite pull it off. Or maybe we did something wrong, really wrong. Maybe we hurt someone else. Maybe we hurt ourselves. Maybe we chose perfection as an unreachable standard, and had to punish ourselves for not hitting the unreachable mark. For whatever reason, somewhere along the way, we realized we didn't like ourselves.

We don't show up at the door step of self-hatred one day out of the blue. There is a path that is followed to get to this point. There are steps along the path that lead us to this place of self-loathing that is in direct contrast to God's view of us. I learned about these steps at the Wellspring School of Ministry from Dr. Art Mathias. They are expanded on in his book, *Biblical Foundations for Freedom*:

Unforgiveness

At some point in time, have you ever discovered or decided that you had not forgiven yourself? Did you choose to replay this offense in your mind rather than forgiving yourself quickly? Over time, the issue seemed to grow, we may have even begun to add "friends" (additional strikes against ourselves) and we just kept it all inside. We berated ourselves that this was only getting worse. Any failure leads to our condemning ourselves for falling short . . . again. Can you relate?

Resentment

The next step along the path is resentment. Once we have gathered offenses against ourselves and have not forgiven ourselves for what we have done, big or small, we begin to resent ourselves. Thoughts in this stage may be "I can't ever do anything right." Or "Mother was right, I'll never amount to anything." Have you ever said things like this to yourself?

Retaliation

After we spend some time resenting ourselves, we decide we have to do something to get back at ourselves. After all, this has gone on too long! Sadly, in this phase we don't just get back at ourselves, we may allow others to get back at us, too! We become defensive any time we feel like someone is accusing us of doing anything wrong. We respond quickly, strongly, and negatively. We do all this to defend the lies we are entertaining in our lives. Have you snapped at anyone in the past week? Can you think of some ways you have snapped at yourself?

Anger

Once we begin to retaliate against ourselves on a regular basis, we progress to self-anger. We don't arrive here overnight. This "stepping stone" along the self-bitterness path can only be reached after a period of time when something has been "simmering and festering just below the surface" for days, weeks, months, or even years. At this point, we don't just dislike a few things about ourselves, we *categorically do not love ourselves at all any longer* (if we ever did). This is a dangerous level to reach. You may know people, or may even be someone yourself, who can't seem to do anything right in her or your own eyes. You may participate in self-loathing and even self-punishing yourself. It becomes a vicious cycle that continues, possibly even to the point of self-murder.

Violence/Murder

People who have reached the stage of self-violence or self-murder are entertaining thoughts of ending their own lives. They may say aloud or to themselves things like, "No one would miss me if I weren't around anymore. In fact, the world would be a better place without me." They have come into agreement with the lies of the enemy that they are not valuable, they are not needed, they will NEVER be good enough no matter how hard they try, no one else really cares about them, and they just don't want to go on anymore.

I'd like to clarify here that we can "murder" ourselves with our words, not only our actions. And, in essence, we can even "murder" others with our words. That whole "Sticks and stones may break my bones, but words will never hurt me" thing is a LIE! With just a few poorly-chosen (and sometimes unintentional) words, we can kill someone's hope, their dreams, undermine their gifting, talents or even abilities. Sometimes, we don't even have to say a word at all. Our body language can say it all. We will dig into the power of our spoken words to others, and to ourselves, in the next chapter. For now, it's time to get some freedom from self-condemnation for you!

As I write this, my heart is heavy for those who may be in the self-violence/self-murder stage even now. It is difficult and uncomfortable to admit, but true, that I have personally been through every single one of these stages earlier in my life. I absolutely BELIEVED the lies that the enemy was constantly feeding me. I am sharing something here I have only shared with a very few people, ever. But I've come to realize it's important for me to share so others may have hope.

When I was in my early twenties, fresh out of college, working 70+ hours a week in the field of child abuse investigation, I was so overwhelmed by my negative beliefs about myself and the circumstances of my life that I planned to take my own life. I had a specific plan, but thankfully I wasn't brave enough to execute it, even though I intended to for several days in a row.

In hindsight, it would have been the most selfish thing I could have ever done. I would never have known my daughter. My life would have been little more than a big tragedy. But the truth was, God had more for me. Thankfully, at some level, deeply buried beneath a lot of pain, I knew that, and I wanted and needed more of God!

Tim and I made some significant life changes (a move, job changes, lifestyle changes, and more) to help me get to a healthier place. It took me over six months to heal from the pain I had felt and to begin to feel joy again. Over time, I began to learn how to address these deep pains, and I am thankful that today it seems surreal to recount that painful season of my life. It's like I'm talking about a different person. In many ways, I am. I bless the Lord for loving me, for not only showing me truth in His Word and for bringing loving people across my path, but for the DRAMATIC way He pursued and wooed me for my healing, and for His glory!

So, if you are anywhere along the path today, may I confidently assure you that there is HOPE! You don't have to progress even one step further. I have an encouraging word for you. I have been where you are, and I know how to get out of that spiral, tail-spin pattern that has been pulling you down for far too long.

Would you believe that you are not solely to blame for those negative thoughts and feelings you have been harboring against yourself? I know, you may feel like you alone have caused all this mess, but that's a lie. And it is a sibling to a whole bunch of other lies that have been fed to you, and that you have come into agreement with.

I've heard that the enemy doesn't know our thoughts, but that he can plant thoughts into our minds. So we all have fleeting thoughts that skip across our minds from time to time that just don't seem to "fit in" with our usual thoughts. Those random, out-of-place thoughts are probably from the enemy. They happen to everyone. We must remember our charge and our authority to "take every thought captive" (2 Corinthians 10:5), meaning that we need to be aware of which thoughts we are agreeing with, which ones we are dwelling on, and which ones we need to kick out of our thinkers.

Yes, we have the power to control our minds. In fact, not only are we *able* to, we are *expected* to take control of our minds. And something that I frequently say out loud is a gentle reminder that "I have the mind of Christ." (1 Corinthians 2:16, ESV) I especially find myself saying this when my mind may feel confused, overwhelmed, or just unsure. I speak it as truth in faith that my own thoughts will come into agreement with it and my mind will clear up. Again, we will spend more time on the power of our spoken words later in this text.

Do you see how these destructive thoughts keep our focus is on ourselves and are not on God? We are making ourselves into some kind of idol that we focus on day and night. We may or may not be having consistent time in God's Word, but much of our thought life is on US, and our shortcomings, our many, many shortcomings.

In much the same way as you began your forgiveness list in chapter five, begin a list of things you need to forgive about yourself.

What are you mad at yourself about? What did you do that you deeply wish you could un-do? What didn't you do that you wish you could go back and get a second chance? What was the topic at your most recent pity party? What part of your body are you obsessed about? Can you forgive yourself for not being perfect? Will you forgive yourself for eating that bag of potato chips? That's right, choosing to forgive is an act of our will. I believe you can.

Any time we come into agreement with a lie that the enemy has planted in our mind, we are in sin. We are basically choosing to agree with what he says about us (condemnation) over what God says about us (love). In a sense, we are calling God a liar when we choose the enemy's lie over God's truth. Let that sink in for a few minutes. To say it another way, when you partner with a lie of the enemy, you are choosing a lie over God's love. The good news is, this agreement can be broken when we renounce (break agreement with) it.

Here's a simple prayer for you to follow along with as you begin to forgive yourself. Remember, it's simple, but it's powerful! Pray through every single specific issue *individually*. Take the time you need to go through this process as thoroughly as possible, but don't rush it. You don't have to have it all listed out and prayed through this week.

In fact, it may take weeks or even months to work through the self-bitterness matters the Father brings to your mind. But this process is worth investing time and emotional energy into. You will likely experience some significant shifts and some intense emotional reactions as you work through your list. That's okay. Embrace the tears and even the snot. Embrace the laughter. It means you're doing the business of getting free from past hurts and past pains. Press into the Father. Listen to what He says to and about you. He loves you. And He wants better for you.

Give yourself permission to cry, to laugh, to sing, to dance, whatever you feel led to do. Freedom creates some cool new activities in us! Embrace them!

Prayer for Release of Self-Bitterness

"Heavenly Father, in the name of Jesus, and as an act of my free will, I confess, repent, and renounce my (specific sin of self-bitterness). I ask you to forgive me for this sin. From my heart, I purpose and choose to forgive myself for this (specific sin). I release myself from any guilt or shame because of this self-bitterness. In the name of Jesus, and by the power of His blood, I cancel Satan's authority over me in this situation. Holy Spirit, heal my heart and reveal your truth to me about this situation."

Listen and record what the Holy Spirit shows you. (Remember, you may have a picture come to mind, or a thought, a different memory, a word, a smell, even a taste or a feeling as you pause and listen to the Father after this prayer.)

After you have prayed through as many of these issues as you have had come to mind, command the spirit of self-bitterness to go, in the name of Jesus. You don't have to raise your voice or stomp. I don't believe the enemy is hard of hearing. But if you want to stomp and snort, go for it!

As you go through this worthwhile, life-changing process, I hope you will begin to experience "Love your neighbor as yourself" in a whole new, loving way. I believe that by so doing we are strengthening not only our physical bodies, but also the Body of Christ which will become healthier and stronger as we choose to be blessed, and to be a blessing to others and to ourselves.

As we conclude this chapter, here's something for you to think about. There is a mounting collection of evidence that suggests autoimmune disorders are related to self-bitterness issues. Think about it. In an autoimmune disorder, the body is supposedly "attacking itself" . . . in many instances the person has been attacking herself for years prior to the development of the autoimmune disorder. So, you may be wondering, "If I have an autoimmune disorder, could it be addressed by applying a healthy dose of self-forgiveness?" Many others have found this to be the case. I pray it will be so for you, too!

Chapter Seven

Choose to Speak Words of Life

Most of us are pretty good at talking. Some of us are pretty good at listening. But I wonder how many really understand the POWER that is within every single word we speak, write, whisper, or even think.

Have you ever considered the value and power of the words you say every day, to others, and to yourself? Would you believe that by changing a few of the words you use, and perhaps by omitting some words from your vocabulary altogether, you could make a visible change in your life and the lives of others around you?

Most of us have two dialogues running inside our minds at any given point of time. One dialogue addresses those around us. The other addresses ourselves. For now we are going to explore the power of our SPOKEN words. In the next chapter, we'll dig deeper into the power of the words we "say" to ourselves, the words that make up our thoughts, and the words we may speak aloud to ourselves (in case you're like me and talk aloud to yourself) ALL of our words are incredibly powerful. But let's begin with the original spoken word.

Creation Was Spoken Into Being

In the first chapter of the book of Genesis, we read the words, "God said" nine different times. Each time, He called into existence something that was not there before. Will you take a moment to let that sink in? When He spoke, He changed things. When He spoke, He created things. WOW!

The first time we read about this is in Genesis 1:3 "And God said, 'Let there be light." (ESV) At that very moment, He spoke something out of nothing. He spoke the creation we see and enjoy into existence. He didn't reach down and take up a handful of sand from the beach and whip it up into something, He merely SPOKE, and things changed. He could have used any other method. But, He CHOSE to speak. (Okay, even though I have taught this many times and have pondered it for several years at the time of this writing, this still gets to me! I am in AWE of His power . . . and the way He chooses to do things!) So what does this suggest? After all, we know we are made in His image. We are like Him in many ways. Might it suggest there is immeasurable power in *our* spoken words, too?

Think about this for a minute: God spoke creation into existence. We are made in His image. We do a lot of things the way He does them. So, have you ever thought about this? Did you know the words you speak can literally change things? Let this revelation sink in and change you as we look at the biblical basis of this concept.

Blessings

Further on in the book of Genesis, we read of another use of the spoken word. In those days, as a patriarch approached the end of his life, it was customary for him to SPEAK a blessing over his oldest son. As Isaac was approaching his death, he called for Esau, his older son, to give him his (Isaac's) blessing. You may be familiar with the part of the story in which Isaac's younger son, Jacob, and his mother, Rebecca, plotted to steal this blessing from Esau so that Jacob could receive it instead of Esau. As the first-born son, Esau was entitled to receive his father's blessing.

This story was an example of deception at its finest! Isaac sent Esau out to gather the ingredients to prepare a special meal for Isaac, whose vision had failed him by this late season in his life. While Esau was gone, Rebecca quickly whipped up a great meal. She disguised Jacob's arms with hairy animal skin, (as Esau was reported to be quite hairy!) so that when Isaac felt Jacob's arms, they would feel like his brother.

Keep in mind that Jacob had already wrangled Esau's birthright from him in a prior lapse of "hangry" judgment on Esau's part. That had been another act of deception in Jacob's life. But that's another chapter. For now, let's see what happened when Jacob presented himself as his brother and asked to receive Isaac's blessing.

Genesis 27:30-40 (NAS) details these events. When elderly Isaac gave the blessing, Jacob, not Esau, was there to receive it. In verse 33 we read of Isaac's reaction at the moment he realized his blessing had gone out from him, but to the *wrong person*! This was no small matter. We read that "Isaac trembled violently . . ." Trembling violently suggests Isaac was very upset! He recognized that the power of his blessing had already left him and it had gone to the wrong person! It wasn't as if he could just take it back and Isaac knew it. It was already out there. The spoken blessing had already gone to work in Jacob's life. AND Isaac could not bestow the same blessing upon Esau.

So, Isaac bestowed a different kind of "blessing" upon Esau. We read the details of it in verses 37-40.

But did you notice that in verse 36 Esau said, "Isn't he rightly named Jacob?" The name Jacob means "He grasps the heel. Supplanter. Underminer." Esau recognized the value of the spoken word. He knew that he had missed out on his father's blessing, to which he was rightly entitled as the older son, and he knew that the meaning of his brother's name was spoken back into him every time it was spoken, every time Jacob heard it. Every time someone spoke the name Jacob, they were speaking supplanter and underminer into him. It's valuable to know the meaning of your name, since that is what is being spoken into your life every time someone speaks your name.

Let's take a moment here to explore this little tidbit before we proceed. Do you know the meaning of your name? Have you ever looked it up? Take a moment to Google the meaning of your name.

For example, my name is spelled uniquely, so you can look at it from two different perspectives:

Diana means "heavenly, divine, luminous, perfect." I'm thankful those are positive words.

But my name is spelled DiAnna, which could mean a double (Di) Anna . . . Anna means favor or grace, so maybe that's why I see so much favor and grace in my life! People all around me are speaking grace and favor into me every time they say my name, and I receive that!

How do you feel about the meaning of your name? I know of woman who legally changed her name as she learned about these principles. As an adult, she came into a relationship with Jesus and felt her name was too cold for the vibrant new life she was given, so she changed it. I'm not suggesting you need to change your name, but I do think it is valuable to be aware of what is being spoken into you every time someone speaks your name.

Will you take a few more moments to look up the names of your spouse, your children, your siblings, and others who are close to you?

Okay, let's keep cruising along here . . . We've talked about the value of our spoken words as blessings. Now let's look at the opposite of blessings and curses.

Curses

We also read of the first curses in the book of Genesis. In the same way as a blessing, a curse in biblical times could not be revoked or changed. Once it was spoken and thus in place, it stood. Here are a few examples.

Genesis 3:14. "So the Lord God said to the serpent, Because you have done this, Cursed are you above all the livestock and all the wild animals." (ESV) Who knows what the serpent may have looked like, or how he may have gotten around before that moment, but we all know that to this day, serpents must slither on their bellies to get anywhere. And they can only slither just so fast before a predator (maybe a country woman with a hoe!) catches up to them.

In Genesis 3:17-19, God said to Adam, "Because you listened to your wife and ate from the tree about which I commanded you, 'You must not eat of it. Cursed is the ground because of you; through painful toil you will eat of it all the days of your life. In pain you shall eat of it all the days of your life; thorns and thistles it shall bring forth for you; and you shall eat the plants of the field. By the sweat of your face you shall eat bread, till you return to the ground, for out of it you were taken; for you are dust, and to dust you shall return." (ESV) There has been a curse on the land ever since that moment. Adam and Eve were soon kicked out of the garden, and life for them was never the same.

The passage above suggests that prior to the Curse, there were no thorns and thistles, but there have been thorns and thistles ever since, and there will be to the end of time. The power of a curse is lasting.

In Genesis 4:11, we read that after killing his brother Abel, Cain was placed under a curse. The ground would no longer yield crops for him. He was to be a restless wanderer on the earth for the remainder of his life.

Generational Curses:

Further along in the Bible, we read of some curses lasting generations. This is a real issue affecting many people even today. While we will not go into this topic in this book, I hope you will take some time to further research curses that last generations and do what is necessary to break off the curses affecting you and your generation so that they will not pass to generations after you. We need to remember our authority as co-heirs with Jesus Christ to powerfully address and even break off tormenting curses in our lives, so that our children won't have to deal with the same ones in their lives.

Here's another side note on this topic. In my work as a Naturopathic Doctor, some people have thought it is funny to refer to me as a "witch doctor." Isn't that a terrible thing to call someone? The very word "witch" suggests a satanic anointing under which I most certainly do not operate. So, I've become very comfortable asking my clients not to refer to me that way, even if they think it's funny. I explain that I take the power of the spoken word seriously and that I don't receive that label or the curse that may be associated with it. And sure, in spite of my requests, I know it still happens from time to time. I'm not responsible for the actions or words of others. But I wonder, how would our world be different if more people understood and harnessed the power within their spoken words?

You can imagine that I was extremely thrilled to discover a provision for an "unjust curse" in Proverbs 26:2. "Like a fluttering sparrow or a darting swallow, an undeserved curse does not come to rest." (NIV) Another translation reads, "An unjust curse will not fall on a righteous man." (The Message) I love that! I am not a witch doctor. I don't deserve the curse that goes along with that terrible name or phrase, and I can feel assured that the associated (and undeserved) curse will not fall on me. Maybe there's a phrase or some other kind of curse in your own life that you can apply this verse to. Will you take a moment to reflect and ask the Holy Spirit to bring to mind any "unjust curses" that may have been spoken to or over you?

Now that we've established the Biblical precedence for blessings and curses, let's bring these principles to today's time. How do we curse others?

Have you ever heard yourself start a statement with one of the following phrases?

"You *always* . . . "

"You *never* . . . "

"You are out of your ever-loving mind!"

"You are crazy if you think . . . "

When we make statements like these, we are speaking curses into those to whom we are directing our comments. The words "always" and "never" are pretty powerful, and I would dare to say each of them is quite overused.

Now really, for example, does anyone ALWAYS leave the toilet seat up? Like, every single time? If so, can we just purpose and choose to forgive them anyway? Maybe we can even go the extra mile and put that toilet seat down to the glory of Jesus? Meanwhile, by not saying "always" we are not placing a curse on them. We can choose instead to bless them.

Or, could it be possible that they NEVER remember to take out the trash on time? Oh sure, maybe they never have up to this point . . . but does that really mean that they never will? If we speak that word *never* over them, we may actually be placing a curse onto them. Again, remember and access the power of forgiveness so that you won't host unconfessed sin that will hold you back from right relationship with them, and from right relationship with our Father. Instead, choose to bless that person.

Have you heard yourself say something like, "You're crazy if you think I am going out into that cold creek!" Is it really possible that we spoke craziness into someone else? Yes, it really is! As you are reading along here, does it seem to you that I may be taking this spoken word thing just a bit too far? I hope not. It's my hope and prayer that you are receiving fresh revelation that the words that you speak are powerful! They are powerful enough to change **things**. They are powerful enough to change **people**. They are powerful enough to change **lives**.

Thankfully, we can use our words to bless others, not only curse them. We have an opportunity to speak, in faith, blessing into the lives of everyone we meet, every single day. Let's think about what that might look like. Because not every blessing will be as dramatic as the one Esau spoke over and into Isaac.

The principle here of the power of our spoken word is so powerful, and so underutilized, that I believe and know from personal experience that when we become intentional about using it for good, then we will begin to see changes in others that previously we could have only hoped or imagined.

Have you ever heard of "calling something out of someone"? I'm not talking about demons or other principalities here, I'm talking about seeing something within someone else that she may not even know about herself, and speaking it into her life. It might look something like this. Let's suppose you have a friend who has a knack for decorating her home. She may not realize that not everyone can quickly create a shiplap wall and then effortlessly coordinate the colors, textures, and furniture in a room in one afternoon. She may even say, "Well, it wasn't anything, really. I just threw a few things together." You have an opportunity here to call out her inner decorator. Your words can affirm her natural giftings, and call her up to recognize that what seems so natural and easy to her, is truly a gift, talent, or ability that not everyone possesses. You see something in her that she doesn't recognize about herself, and you call it out of her. You are speaking a blessing into her life, words of life, and that blessing doesn't stop with her.

Let's continue this example just awhile longer. You already told her that she has a knack for creating a warm, inviting space while resourcefully using things she already has around the house. She may graciously accept this as a compliment, or she may shrug off your words but in either case, you planted a seed into her life by the words you spoke and that seed will sprout. Maybe a few days later she finds herself visiting with a young friend who is getting ready to set up her first apartment. Her friend isn't sure how to go about decorating or making this new space feel like home or comfortable, so your friend offers to come over to help her get settled in, and she shares her gift of decorating and hospitality with this younger friend. Together, they create a space that is warm and cozy. And like her own home, she invites people to linger and enjoy relationships. Do you see how the words you spoke affirmed something in your friend that went on to bless other people?

I've long used the principle of speaking in faith with my clients. One of the most rewarding facets of health consulting is that glimmer of hope in someone's eyes after a period of time when they felt hopeless about their health. Once we've determined a course of action to help them reach their health goals, I make sure to assure them that I believe they can and will follow through on this new course to better health. Did you catch that? It was kind of subtle, but I don't want you to miss it. I speak faith into them when I assure them that I know they CAN and WILL follow through on their new health program. They hear my voice say, "I know you can do this." or "It won't be easy, but you are worth the effort." I am also speaking other things into them such as "You are going to love the way you feel when you come back in a couple weeks." I am calling out a healthier self that is already within them. I am planting hope and expectation that things will be better in the future than they have been in the past. And guess what? They follow through and they experience results.

Practice speaking a new thing into your children or your spouse. In the natural, you may not see them fulfilling the potential you know the Father has placed within them. You may see a quality within them that they have not yet discovered about themselves, so use the power of your words to call out their greatness.

When I first met my husband Tim, he had been in a relationship where he felt beaten down emotionally. When we met, his self-confidence was low. He had been hurt, but I saw a greatness within him. I began to encourage him. I believed in him and I let him know it. These words of life lifted his spirits elevated the way he operated in his giftings.

After we had been married about five years, Tim yielded to a calling on his life to go into ministry, but he didn't believe he could talk in front of people. I encouraged him to follow God's leading and affirmed the leadership qualities I saw within him. It's difficult to imagine now, over twenty years later, that he ever had any reservations about talking in front of large groups. He has pastored three churches and helped start over sixteen cowboy churches across the state of Arkansas. I believe God used my words to encourage Tim to walk into his purposes. We have that kind of power in the words we speak.

And yes, one of the lives your spoken words change is your very own! We will dig into that topic in our next chapter. But for now, will you begin to pay closer attention to the words you speak? Will you share this material with a close friend or spouse and ask them to help you hear the words you speak to others? (If they want extra credit, they can even begin listening to the words you speak aloud to yourself.)

Chapter Eight

Take Every Thought Captive

Do you ever talk to yourself? If you are a female, you probably instantly responded "Yes!" to that question. But if you are a male, there is at least a 50/50 chance that you thought something like, "Ummm, no, I've not even thought about talking to myself. What would I even say?" And while the men are thinking those statements, the women may have already had three mini conversations with ourselves! Right?

We've heard that men speak about 10,000 words a day and women speak about 25,000 words every day. It just makes sense that women talk to ourselves, who else is gonna listen to all those words? But seriously, it is worth every moment of your valuable time to not only pay attention, but really DIG INTO this topic of the power of the words we speak to ourselves. Because sometimes the things we say to ourselves are not very kind. I know you know what I'm talking about here. Can you honestly say that there is ANYONE else you talk to the same way you talk to yourself? It's doubtful.

As I've shared with you about my past, you may know that I spent my first forty-two years pretty much "hating on" myself. It usually seemed like I couldn't do anything "good enough" or that I should always be able to do more. I focused way too much on my flaws and was virtually incapable of pointing out positive qualities I possessed. These perceived shortcomings, flaws, and criticisms were the topics of many of my *internal* conversations.

But I would also reiterate these internal beliefs with my spoken words. I'm going to list a few statement openers below. See if any of these resonate with you.

"That drives me crazy!"

"You're making me crazy!"

"You are driving me nuts!"

"I could never . . . "

"I would never . . . "

"That makes me sick."

"I always . . . "

"You're killing me. . . "or, "It's killing me. . ."

And a former favorite, "One of these days I'm gonna…"

As it turns out, one of these days is none of these days . . . and our body will not be bluffed by a conflict in our intentions (what we intend to do) and what we SAY we will do. It always believes our WORDS!

Think about it, your voice is the voice your body hears more than anyone else's. So, your voice is more believable to your body than anyone else's voice is. Which means, if your mother or husband always tells you that you are smart, beautiful, kind, and loving, but at the same time, you are constantly telling yourself you are stupid, fat, ugly, and a total crab then who are you more likely to believe? Or to put that question another way, whose words will have the most effect on your actions? Think about it. How is this resonating with you?

You may be noticing that I am separating you from your body in the statements above. Have you ever thought of the two of you as separate? Your body is just your lifetime hotel, but it is not YOU. We talked in chapter one about our body being a temple of the Holy Spirit, but it is a temple . . . a dwelling place . . . IT is not who you ARE. Oh sure, when people think of us, and even when we see ourselves, our body is what we see, it is recognizable, and it is closely associated *with* us. But it's our soul, which is made up of our mind, will, emotions along with our spirit man and THAT's who we really ARE.

So, as a separate entity from who we ARE, our body actually reacts and responds to our spoken words as if they are gospel truth every time! Alright ladies, this means that every time you speak the words "I am so fat" – your body hears that and puts processes into motion to carry out that very statement into truth. Seriously? Yes, seriously.

Every time you say, "That makes me so sick!" your body hears those words and puts literal sickness into play. Have you ever noticed that you may fall ill after having an emotional spike? It happens – and it happens too often! Please pay attention to what you say. I guarantee your words are affecting your physical health, emotional health, and even spiritual health way more than you had ever imagined. And the great news is this, it works both ways!

My examples thus far have been negative ones, but you can work this to your advantage with just as much certainty. For example, we can speak healing into our own lives as well, such as saying, "I am healthy and strong. Every cell in my body is healing." You know what? That is a true statement. Your body's default is healing. It is constantly in a state of healing and repair. That's how God made our bodies to work!

In Ephesians 4:29, we are exhorted by the Apostle Paul, "Do not let any unwholesome talk come out of your mouths, but only what is helpful for building others up according to their needs, that it may benefit those who listen." (NIV) Our words have the power to build up others, which presumes the opposite is true and they can also tear down others – and ourselves.

Have you already thought of at least one way that you tear yourself down with your words? Maybe you don't want to think of yourself as tearing you down, maybe you prefer to lighten it up and realize that you are just holding yourself back. Either way, can we agree that the moment we realize that we have been cursing ourselves with our words is a "Hallelujah moment"! Yes indeed, Hallelujah that we realize we are off track. We realize that we are not spurring ourselves onto greater things, rather we are keeping ourselves from being all that God has designed us to be. That's a sobering thought, isn't it?

When we recognize that we have been agreeing with a lie, something that isn't true, we see that is sin AND we have an opportunity to deal with it right then and there!

Let's break agreement with these lies and repent to our loving Heavenly Father for believing the lies in the first place. It's likely that until now you may not have realized that believing these lies has held you back from God's best for your life.

Will you take some time to create a list of the negative things you speak into your own life? We both know it happens. Maybe you missed a turn on the way to work today and proceeded to blurt out a string of special language. Maybe you forgot to sign your daughter's field trip permission slip, again. Maybe you are critical of the "bat wings" under your arms. Maybe you have spoken negatively about some body part. Will you write it all down? This isn't designed to condemn you. You know that. This is a process that may be uncomfortable, after all, you probably haven't done this before, but it will help you get freedom from the pain it causes you. It also helps you see the Father's perspective on the situation. He loves you. He wants you to love yourself. Really.

Here's a repentance prayer you can use as a guide to help you address each and every one of the ways you have been condemning yourself through your words.

Heavenly Father, forgive me for cursing myself when I say (the specific words you say). I purpose and choose to forgive myself from my heart. In the name of Jesus, I cancel Satan's authority over me in this sin and command the tormentors assigned to me to go now.

Holy Spirit, heal my heart and show me the truth about this situation.

Listen.

What happened after your prayed that? What did the Holy Spirit show you? Isn't that a precious gift He has given you? He loves you so much! And He wants you to love yourself, too!

Over the next couple weeks, I hope you will continue the process of really paying attention to what you say to yourself. Ask the Holy Spirit to guard your every spoken word this week. Will you give Him permission to bring those words to your attention? Can you expect Him to do a wonder work in the words you speak and the way you speak them? Would you agree with me in asking Him for the following?

Holy Spirit, help me take captive every thought I have this week. Show me the ways I have cursed myself, or others, through my words. Show me the truth about each situation you reveal to me. Help me be a blessing, not a curse, to myself, to others, and for you. I bless you, Lord, and thank you for the work you are doing in my life!

Chapter Nine

Fear Not

You may not consider yourself a fearful person. It seems like most people deny feeling fear, but they speak it, and even walk it out more often than they realize.

Can we wade into the waters of how fear is damaging your life and how it is holding you back? Did you notice that I didn't pussyfoot around and say that fear might be affecting you? Because whether you are a woman or a man, no matter how brave you may believe yourself to be, you are being affected by fear. In this chapter, I'll show you how it is wreaking havoc on your life and what it takes to get rid of it.

Would you describe yourself as a worrier? Do you ever feel like if you don't worry about something, who will? Do you hear yourself say any of the following?

"I'm worried that . . . "

"I'm afraid if I _____ then _____ will happen."

Or the ever-popular, "What if..." Maybe we say, "What if something goes wrong?" or "What if _____ happens?"

When I was in grade school, I was introduced to the saying, "Who died and made you boss?" Did you ever hear that? When we allow ourselves to worry about something, it's kinda like someone died and we became the boss. Do you follow me on that? It's as if by worrying, we believe that we will somehow be able to, in some nebulous way that really makes absolutely no sense, change the outcome of whatever situation we are worrying about. Have you ever been able to change the outcome of something just by worrying about it? Probably not. But rest assured, your worry was not without consequence. We will talk more about that later. But let's spend a bit more time on the "worry monster" before we move along.

Have you heard some of these phrases about worry?

"Worry is just faith in the devil."

"Worry never robs tomorrow of its sorrow – it only snatches today's joy."

And of course, there's everybody's favorite song, "Don't Worry, Be Happy".

I don't want to assume you know how fear or worry is currently tormenting you, so let me describe a woman in fear below.

We all know her. She's a worrier. She's a control freak.

She *seems* nervous. All. The. Time. She FEELS nervous. All. The. Time. From the time she awakens until the time she finally shuts off her overly-chattery mind in the wee hours of the night, she feels wired, but tired. She may know she feels unsettled, or she may just attribute it to "nervous energy" or even excitement for her life. She's fearful. She's constantly thinking of all the "What if's".

She's uncomfortable being alone or being quiet, but having to be alone AND quiet at the same time is just unbearable. It makes her feel uneasy. She doesn't like it. She can't stand it! She can't be in the car alone without the radio on. She can't be home alone without the TV or music playing, or both at the same time! She doesn't really think anything of this, it seems normal to her. There's no time for stillness in her busy, busy life! And if her schedule eases up for a season, she will find or create new things to keep her busy. She will join a new group, sign up her kids for a new sport, or even volunteer at church or a non-profit, just to stay in busy-mode. Stillness is scary. While uncomfortable, being busy is familiar. The familiarity of being busy, while uncomfortable, is less scary than the unknown of stillness.

Speaking of being in the car, when she and her husband go somewhere with the family, she has to drive. She has to drive because this way she can control what happens. This way *she* won't hit anything. This way they won't end up getting lost. This way she can be sure they don't get a speeding ticket, have an accident, and no one will get hurt. She won't have to be angry with her husband if he was driving and anything happened to her precious children. She's able to control all of this by driving instead of trusting someone else who is perfectly capable of handling the task at hand, driving.

She feels overwhelmed by the many responsibilities and roles she fulfills on a daily basis. There is no such thing as "down time". She craves time off, but doesn't know what to do when it comes, because it is too uncomfortable and unfamiliar to have time to relax, recharge, and refocus. Plus, what if during that brief time away from her office someone discovers that she doesn't really have it all together? What if someone finds out that she isn't really as perfect as she seems? What if...

Does any of this seem familiar to you? It does to me. I was this woman for my first 42 years! Yes, I still drive from time to time when my family is all loaded up, but now it is related to avoiding car sickness. (We live in the Ozark Mountains where roads are more like some roller coasters, lots of curves and hills!) Now I love it when my husband or someone else drives. I don't have to be in control. I can just sit back and enjoy the ride. There are so many things you don't see when you are driving. And I don't feel the weight of controlling the whole world on my shoulders anymore. Frankly, my shoulders were never designed to bear that weight anyway, and neither were yours.

So, what does being a control freak or a perfectionist have to do with fear? WHY does someone feels the need to control or to be perfect? She needs to control because she is afraid of what will happen if she isn't in control. She deludes herself with the idea that she is in control in the first place, which is just a big fat lie.

She isn't in control at all. She just thinks she is. It's a double whammy, she is acting from fear and she is agreeing with a lie.

Often, she feels like she needs to be perfect. I once told Bailey that my favorite color was "perfect." Perfect? I have ridden this horse before, for a long time! Perfectionism is a trap. We strive to be something that doesn't even exist…because we are afraid. When I say perfection doesn't exist, there is only one exception that I know of, that is in the person of Jesus Christ. Only He is perfect. The rest of us are all flawed mortals.

Not one of us is or will be perfect this side of heaven. So, may I share a freeing suggestion with you? Quit trying to be perfect. You will only wear yourself out and miss out on so many great things happening in your life. When we are constantly striving for the elusive "perfect" we are always waiting for that next big thing. We are waiting for things to be better. We are working toward getting all our acts together. And we often miss out on the here and now because we are busy striving for something yet to come.

Besides, when our focus is always on the future, we are setting ourselves up for fighting anxiety. The future holds a lot of unknowns. If we feel a strong need to be in control, the unknowns of the future will feel very scary, and we are likely to become quite anxious.

Remember when I said that your worry is not without consequence? Here's the rest of the story. When we have a fearful feeling, you know the one where there is a distinct tightening in your chest or throat, maybe your arms, hands, or your feet tingle maybe your heart quickens, you may even feel short of breath for a moment . . . yes, *that* feeling. When we have a feeling like that, whether it is in reaction to a thought, a memory, or even a perceived (possible) threat, our body responds. Specifically, our autonomic nervous system signals our adrenal glands to secrete epinephrine (adrenaline) and/or cortisol to respond to the stressor. This allows our pupils to dilate to take in more information and our other senses are heightened. Then our heart beats faster to allow better blood flow to all our extremities and then our body is ready to respond to the threat! ***Even if the threat is only imagined.*** Even if the threat is only in our mind via the "family tradition" of worry.

A helpful analogy to our body's stress response is a fire truck. Once it is dispatched, the lights, bells and whistles all go off! It rushes out of the fire station bay full speed ahead! It goes out "all guns a blazin'!" Every. Single. Time. It doesn't matter if the fire truck is headed to a five-alarm, fully-involved house fire or if it is being dispatched to help Mrs. Smith's cat come down out of the tree, it responds the very same way. Every. Single. Time. So it is with our body's response to any stressor, whether it is real (we just dodged a near-miss car accident), remembered (remember when the ex filed for divorce), or perceived (what if my child doesn't come home this time), our body responds the same exact way. Over time, these reactions can create an inflammatory response in the body that can look like food sensitivities, (yes there really have been people who used to have food sensitivities "lose" them after praying through fears!) or swollen, painful joints, or a host of other situations where it appears the body is "attacking itself" and more.

Now, while I'm speaking against being a perfectionist control freak, I'm not suggesting you give up on excellence. There is a difference between the elusive (non-existent) perfection and the attainable excellence. Without getting way off track here and chasing a major rabbit, let me reference Philippians 4:8 to define excellence:

"Finally, brethren, whatever is true, whatever is honorable, whatever is right, whatever is pure, whatever is lovely, whatever is of good repute, if there is any excellence and if anything worthy of praise, dwell on these things." (NAS)

All the good stuff is in excellence . . . but I didn't notice the word "perfect" here. Excellence requires us to do our best, with the resources we have in our hands right this very minute, to accomplish our purpose TODAY. Tomorrow's purpose may be a bit different, but we can't usually predict just what that will be, so let's be satisfied with accomplishing today's purpose with excellence.

Now that we have clarified the difference between perfection and excellence, let's get back to what fear has to do with all this anyway.

In 2 Timothy 1:7 we read: "For God has not given us a spirit of fear, but of power, and of love, and a sound mind." (NKJV) Wow! Talk about a content-rich verse. I love this verse and share it often. It has so many facets that it can be used in many contexts. For this moment, though, let me ask you this, if God hasn't given us a spirit of fear, then who has?

Have you ever thought about this verse in that way? I hadn't either. If God hasn't given us a spirit of fear, then who has? Maybe fearful patterns were set into our lives by well-meaning parents. Perhaps we model our worry after our mothers. After all, don't all good mothers worry? (Do you see how subtly these detrimental thoughts can be planted into us?)

Maybe well-meaning friends planted the seeds of fear into our lives, "Don't you know that others will think you are weird if you dress like that? Or if you eat that? Or if you do that?" Or, "All the cool kids are going to this party. If you don't go, they'll think you are a baby." This is really related to a fear of man and a spirit of rejection, which we will deal with more thoroughly in the next chapter.

Our own life experiences can create fear or a fearful reaction. If we have been in a car accident, we may become fearful of driving or of riding in a car. If we have a miscarriage, we may become fearful of having another one and losing another baby. Remember how our own voice is the most believable to our body? Take some time now to reflect on and recall fear-based words you have spoken over your own life. Ask Holy Spirit to bring to mind things you have said about yourself, your life, or fears you have entertained.

Even other people's experiences can create fear in us. We may see a tragic story on the news and begin to imagine if that same thing happened to us or to one of our loved ones. Oh my goodness, how awful that would be . . . and then, what if that happened to me? Did you catch it? "What if" strikes again! Don't go there. Be aware of your thoughts, then take them captive. Don't allow them to take you on a wild goose chase and tangle you up in fear!

The bottom line, and ultimate answer is this: Any and all fear we feel comes from the enemy. Let that soak in. Again, if God hasn't given us a spirit of fear, then fear comes from the enemy. The one who seeks to steal, kill and destroy your life is accomplishing his life-destruction mission by using fear in your life. Why would he do that? Likely because he is fearful himself.

He knows his future. Drowning in a sea of fire forever sounds scary. So why not try to drag you down with the very feeling of fear that is tormenting him? I say NO! I will not agree with the lies of the enemy. He feeds us lies to defeat us. He feeds us lies hoping we will believe them, (which is a sin because then we are not agreeing with God's truth) and he feeds us lies because when we believe and agree with them, he gets to torment us right here and now with fear – no waiting for eternity!

When I think of fear, I think of it as an evil, tormenting spirit. Wouldn't you agree? You can be cruising along just fine, then you have a fleeting thought and BOOM! Just like that fear is on the scene. In that moment you have a choice to make. Will you agree with the fearful thought? Or will you command it to leave you?

If you choose to come into agreement with a fearful thought, which is a lie, then you are choosing to disagree with God's truth. He didn't give you a spirit of fear. Remember? No matter what the thought is, if it creates a feeling of fear in you, it's a lie. Will you agree with it or not? The choice is yours. If you don't agree with it, a simple technique I have used is to say aloud, "In the name of Jesus, I command the spirit of fear to go, now." And guess what, just like that the fear must leave. It can't stay in the presence of Holy Jesus. The power of His name forces fear to leave. Yes, as co-heirs with Christ we have the authority to command principalities, so use your authority and take care of business.

Note: *Something to keep in mind is this . . . if there are other people around you who may not be on the same spiritual page as you, you do not have to shout this from the rooftops. While you must speak it aloud, it can be quietly whispered under your breath if need be. I do not believe principalities can read our thoughts, so we must speak aloud so they will hear us. Whispering is just as effective as shouting. In my personal experience, I have not found principalities (tormenting spirits) to be hard of hearing. Once I utter the command, they must flee.*

So that's how you deal with current issues of fear: command the spirit of fear to leave in the powerful name of Jesus. But, what about all those fearful thoughts you may have entertained for years? That's right, we have been through enough of this work together that you know to get your list-making skills warmed up.

In the same way you have done before, begin a list of the fears or fearful thoughts that come to mind. It doesn't matter if you only had the thought once, or if it has been a lifestyle thought pattern for you, write it down. Remember, place no judgment on yourself about the matter. Pray and ask Holy Spirit to reveal and bring to mind all the fearful thoughts and feelings you can possibly recall. He will. He wants to help you through this process. He desires freedom, *complete* freedom for you.

Once you feel like your list is complete for the time being, begin to pray through each and every individual fear issue and write down what the Holy Spirit shows you is truth in that matter. I love the way He is waiting right now to minister to your heart. He so loves you and desires freedom for your life. He desires to replace fear with peace, truth, and love. These are all qualities that He possesses in abundance and He desires to infuse into your life, not just in chintzy amounts, but in vast abundance. Will you let Him do this powerful work that only He can do? Will you allow Him to begin to change you? Did you know that, as you begin to pray through your fear list, you may literally notice a change in your countenance? You may notice those vertical lines between your eyes begin to soften or even disappear. You may notice your eyes become softer and brighter. You will definitely notice a new lightness in your spirit. You will feel a sense of peace you couldn't even imagine before, and there may be other physical manifestations of healing as well.

Many people have experienced healing that is beyond medical justification by praying through these kinds of issues. I am only one of many such people. And I hope you will become one of us, too. Get ready to get started on your list and start praying through it. Because remember, "Nothing happens until we pray."

As you begin to pray through these matters, also heighten your awareness of what you are saying, thinking, and believing. Become more aware of how you are choosing to use different words. There may be some phrases you completely omit from your personal language, such as "I'm afraid," or "I'm worried."

For now, let's get started on your list of fears. As with the other lists, be as specific as possible. List each fear separately and pray through each individual experience or situation. Resist the temptation to bundle several experiences together. Take the time to go through each one individually. This process is too valuable to try to find a short cut. Your future and your generations are at stake here. Take the time. Enjoy the journey!

Once you feel like your list is complete, pray the following prayer for each, specific experience.

Heavenly Father, forgive me for believing or agreeing with the fear of (name the specific fear situation). I purpose and choose to forgive myself for believing and coming into agreement with this lie. I cancel the enemy's authority over me in this situation because it is forgiven. Holy Spirit, show me the truth about this situation.

Listen and write down what the Holy Spirit reveals to you.

Oh how I love, love, love this process! Bless the Lord for His great love for YOU!

After you feel like you've pretty much finished up working through your list to the best of your recollection, say aloud, *"In the name of Jesus, I command the spirit of fear to go now."* Use that same powerful but brief prayer anytime and anywhere you feel sneaky fear trying to edge back into your life. It has no place with you.

Chapter Ten

Play for an Audience of One

Let's dig into something called the "Fear of Man." Have you ever heard that phrase before? I'm not talking about feeling afraid of men or women. The "Fear of Man" means that we are, in any way, afraid of what men or women, or anyone else for that matter, may THINK of us, if we do a certain thing, dress a certain way, drive a certain kind of car, wear certain kinds of clothes, eat certain kinds of foods, speak to our children in certain ways, and the list could go on and on of "certain" things. One thing is certain, if we are more concerned about what OTHER PEOPLE **think** about us than what our loving Creator and Heavenly Father **knows** about us, we will surely be missing out on some pretty awesome sauce happenings and experiences in our lives!

Uh oh! Did you just read that last paragraph and think, for even a second, "Well, I can skip this chapter because this is not a problem for me"? Hmmmm . . . okay, then let's look at this a different way.

Let me share with you a few things about myself that you may or may not know already. *Pay close attention to any thoughts or feelings you may have as you read through some of this information.* Those little twinges will give you a clue to where your own Fear of Man may be hiding in your life.

I have been married to my husband for over 26 years at the time of this writing. For almost 19 of those years, we have been church planters and actively involved in the pastorate of three different churches that we have personally been involved in starting. We are Christians in active vocational ministry. As a result of the decision to serve in this way, we have sacrificed in ways I could never have imagined before we left for seminary in January 1994. We have lost relationships (in varying degrees – some just aren't the same as they were before, others hardly exist anymore, and some are completely severed), from very close family members to disgruntled "church hoppers" on a pretty regular basis for the past 20 plus years.

We have gone without things that money can buy, telling our daughter year after year, "This is going to be a skinny Christmas, Bailey." She came to understand that meant she wouldn't get that big present she really wanted, but she would have to be satisfied with whatever we could afford. And she has gone without worldly things more times than not. We always had what we needed, but for many years we rarely got to enjoy things we wanted. (Does this make you feel uncomfortable? Do you find yourself thinking, "Goodness, why don't you just get a normal job and get on with it? What must people think of you?" Maybe you are thinking along these lines, maybe not, but let's keep moving.)

And let me ask you a "what if" question: what if we had decided at some point that it just wasn't worth it? (Honestly, I decided that very thing many a Saturday night as my husband worked into the wee hours finishing his sermon for the next morning.) What if it became more important to us what others thought of us than the calling we knew was placed on our lives? What if we instead sacrificed what God had called us to so we wouldn't disappoint our loved ones? So we wouldn't have to move away from our families? So we could be more like the other people at our church? So people in our churches wouldn't get upset with us? So we could enjoy nice things? So we could take some much-needed time off to restore our own relationships?

What if we were more interested in pleasing others than in pleasing our God?

About 10 years ago I decided to begin studying natural health for the purpose of sharing life-giving principles with others through natural means provided through God's creation for the blessing and healing of our lives, physically, mentally and even emotionally. Many of my friends, church members, family members, and pretty much everyone else I knew at the time seemed to think that was "interesting" – but many weren't really in agreement with my beliefs about the value of taking the time to learn about how God has provided for our healing in his creation.

Many still don't share my strong convictions that alternative/ complementary approaches to health are more life-giving than just stuffing down symptoms with a prescription medication that comes with a long list of potentially harmful side effects from dry mouth to death. If you are okay with that risk for your health issue, then more power to you, but if there is possibly a natural, life-blessing remedy for whatever ails me or my family, I'd like the opportunity to exhaust all other options before taking a medication that may have long-term damaging effects.

How are you feeling as you read this? Are you feeling your blood pressure rise a bit? Maybe you are thinking that I'm narrow-minded? You may find yourself wanting to debate me on some controversial issue such as vaccinations, alternative cancer care, or something else. Do you feel that way?

"What if" I let the way you might be thinking hold me back from pursuing THIS call on my life? "What if" I didn't put myself out there to serve clients in this field because some might think I am weird, non-traditional, un-Christian, or even radical? That would be me allowing the Fear of Man to influence me instead of listening to the Father who has called me to this work.

As I write, Bailey is in her senior year of high school. It's an exciting season of transition for our family, as it is for all families who have a senior at home. Since this is our tenth year of homeschooling, we are feeling emotions we couldn't have imagined ten years ago. What?! Did I just say we homeschool? Did I say that out loud? Why in the world would we homeschool an only child? Don't we know she needs to be socialized? Don't we understand the social isolation that comes from being an only child? (That's a whole different topic, isn't it?!) And what about the potential social isolation that comes from being a preacher's kid (PK)? But then to add insult to injury, we decided that after second grade we would further "isolate" our only child/PK by homeschooling her?! Oh, have mercy!

Don't think for two seconds we haven't had those conversations a few times – but possibly worse yet are the conversations we don't have, because some people will just judge from afar and not allow us to share our personal convictions and reasons for the decisions we have made. But, does it really matter if we have the opportunity to defend ourselves or not? No, no it doesn't. It doesn't matter one iota! Because we are playing to an audience of ONE. And He knows our hearts, our thoughts, our desires, and the calling He's placed on our lives. No, our callings are not the same as anyone else's, but it is incumbent upon us to be faithful to what we are called to do and be.

I could probably go on about how non-mainstream my life may look to others. But I think you've heard enough with the facts that we are Christians in ministry, who have an only child – whom we homeschool, and I am a Doctor of Naturopathy. Do you think there are people who disagree with our choices? Yes. Do you think there are people who may judge us? Absolutely! *Do you think that it is easier to go along with the way everyone else is going?* If so, there it is. **That** is the Fear of Man!

When we make decisions that prevent, avoid, or minimize our possible conflict with others, what is really happening? We may be holding back from something God has called us to – or from – because we are afraid what others will or might think. We are afraid of man. (Dramatic pause here . . . . powerful "I get it" moment!)

Do you see it now? We are afraid of being judged by someone else. We are afraid they will compare US to themselves and somehow we will fall short. We are afraid because we believe (the lie) that what they think actually matters!

Fear of Man is NOT the fear of what a man may do to us. It isn't even fear of what a man may say about us, it is a fear of what someone may think of us. And at the moment when we allow what man *may* think about us to become more important than what God knows about us, we have made man an idol. We have made man more important than God. We have elevated man over God . . . and that is sin.

So what do we say when sin is revealed in our lives? "Hallelujah!" It's a hallelujah moment when sin is revealed because that means that now we are at a point when we can DEAL WITH IT! We can call it what it is, sin, and we can ask for the Father's forgiveness, forgive ourselves, and move on in freedom!

Fear of Man is a huge issue in our culture. It's nothing short of idolatry. And today is the day you can begin to get free from the way it is holding you back, holding you down, and keeping you from finally stepping into some of the bold things you have felt Holy Spirit calling you into for a very long time. You know exactly what I'm talking about, don't you? That still small voice inside that you have hushed for too many years. That God-sized dream that you have shoved back down inside time and again because seriously, what would people think?

It's my hope and prayer that as you are reading this, the Holy Spirit has been ministering a fresh boldness, confidence and strength into you. I believe that as you are reading this you are literally feeling stronger than you have in a long, long time. You are beginning to see possibilities you hadn't considered before. I believe that as you pray through the Fear of Man strongholds in your own life, the Holy Spirit will begin to reveal to you new creative strategies to propel you to the next level of accomplishing the purposes He has for your life. I am excited for you!

But the stronghold known as Fear of Man is tricky. And the power of our God is stronger! Truth is stronger than a lie every time. This chapter's homework is going to be a bit different than previous chapters. No "make a list" page here. This time you will need to press in deeper. You may need to listen longer. You will ask the Holy Spirit to reveal to you, over the course of the next couple or few weeks, ALL the ways you have held back in your life because of what someone else *might* think, say, or even do about something you have said, thought, or even done.

I do think it is a good idea to write down what the Holy Spirit is showing you. That's the power of our testimony! But this area won't be as cut and dried as the previous "list" areas of bitterness, self-bitterness, and fear. This issue has likely infiltrated multiple areas of your life. You will probably be going through your day as usual when you feel a prompting and realize you just had a thought or feeling related to a Fear of Man. Take a quick moment to jot down that revelation realization. Then proceed through your day – until the next "ah ha moment" when you'll jot down the revelation and keep on cruising.

During this process, consider either keeping a page of notes on your phone, or carrying a small note pad in your purse or pocket so you are ready to capture these thoughts at a moment's notice, no matter where you go. It only takes a few seconds to jot down enough information to recall the details of the situation later. Take the time to do this work. It's worth it. You are worth it.

If possible, at the end of each day, set aside some time when you can be alone and quiet to talk with and listen to the Holy Spirit about what He showed you earlier in the day. I strongly encourage you to write down what he shows you about every little thing – or big thing! These matters have been on His mind for a long time. He is thrilled that they are now on your mind, too! He definitely has something He wants to show you about each lie you have been believing.

Remember, this isn't a smackdown session! God isn't waiting to thump you. This is a powerful time of reconciliation between you and the Creator of the universe! He is wooing you ever closer to His heart through this process. He loves you like crazy! He desires all the best for you. And He has plans and purposes for you that will bless others, if you will yield to Him.

Oh, and I want to tell you "the rest of the story" about a couple things I mentioned earlier. Too often people are reluctant to step into what God has for them because they are afraid of what they will have to give up. Some people are resistant to serving in ministry (in any capacity) because they don't want to be poor, or "different," or whatever it is that's hard for them to imagine.

For every single thing I have given up in the past, God has generously replaced it with something of greater value. He has lavishly redeemed (and is still redeeming) every hurt, loss, and discomfort I have experienced. He has provided vacations where we were able to get away as a family in some amazingly beautiful far-away places and hear His voice, reconnect with one another, and refresh our health.

Through His generous provision, Bailey has had some pretty spectacular gifts through the years! And I'll go ahead and add that she is one well-adjusted, God-lovin', beautiful-inside-and-out young lady! She has seen His dramatic provision in ways that most of her peers can hardly imagine. She has seen His loving touch heal people physically time and time again. She has come to expect healing. She is learning to listen to Him and she knows she can trust Him for her best.

While homeschooling may seem a bit odd by some standards, He has used our availability to bless others, draw them to Him, take them deeper in Him, experience His powerful healing touch, comfort hearts, knit hearts, and I could go on and on and on. Ministry can be tough. It is warfare, after all. But as we have learned and applied the principles I am sharing with you, we have become more effective warriors.

Press in. Dig deep. And don't give up until you have heard Him speak to your heart, your mind, your will, and your emotions.

Until you move on, enjoy hearing from God and experiencing newfound freedoms!

Chapter Eleven

Rejection is a Secret Saboteur

Let's move on to the issue of rejection. In some ways, it's closely related to the Fear of Man. If we feel apprehensive about what others may think about us, we may subconsciously hold ourselves back from pursuing what we KNOW is God's design for us. It may feel a lot like fear when we feel rejected by others. It may keep us from jumping in with both feet and never looking back, oh no, because that might feel too scary. Instead, we stay safely on the shore of where we (think we) KNOW what others will think, and we (think we) KNOW they will approve of our intentions, actions, and plans. We don't experience the glory He has purposed for us, but at least we are not risking possible rejection.

Okay, so let's start off by defining rejection. It can mean different things to different people in different contexts, so let's set a common language for this term we'll dig into during this chapter.

Webster's Dictionary defines the verb rejection as "to refuse to accept or consider, to throw off...to repel...to repulse." For the most part, we will focus on that first part, "to refuse to accept" as our primary definition of rejection. With that being clarified, you may wonder, "Where does rejection come from?"

Let's start way back at the beginning of our lives, while we are still in the womb. Do you know if you were a "planned" baby? Or were you a "surprise?" Believe it or not, a small seed of rejection could have been placed into you beginning way back then.

For example, I was born just 10 months after my parents wed. Do you think they planned for that? I don't think so. I've heard my mom say that they had planned to wait about five years before starting a family. She was only 19 years old when she married my daddy. They were living with my grandmother at the time, just getting started in their new life together. A baby probably wasn't on their agenda at that time. But they both always seemed quite happy to have me and they had my younger sister just two and a half years later. She seemed super welcome, too! So it's not as if my parents rejected me just because I was born sooner than they may have planned.

I'm not sure what you believe about what all happens in the womb, when life begins, or a host of other things. And, at one point, I didn't give much consideration to these possibilities myself. But over time, through both reading more about this subject and working with clients who come from all kinds of early life situations, I have developed a strong respect and acknowledgement for what happens inside the womb. I believe that the moment conception occurs, life has begun. And I believe that the developing embryo and fetus can sense mom's emotions (via hormonal "couriers" and developing ears) and that the baby inside is affected by mom's food choices, drug use, alcohol use, and absolutely everything else that is going on around her. The growing fetus hears mom's voice and receives words spoken into it, over it, and about it all through its time in the womb.

That's why newborn babies make and hold eye contact with their daddies and mommies, and other voices they heard while in the womb. Those voices are familiar to them. The babies recognize them, not because they've heard them since birth; they've heard them since shortly after conception.

The baby hears what is being spoken about it. Remember how much power there is in the spoken word? So the baby hears all that is being spoken about it, around it, and near it. I believe development and growth are affected by traumas of any sort experienced by mom or baby during gestation. And guess what, the cells within the body never forget a single trauma. Every past trauma, emotional hurt, exposure to a virus, and a host of other issues are coded into the molecular makeup for each person. So, it's not beyond the scope of possibility that a developing embryo sensed a moment of surprise rejection upon mom's discovery that she is pregnant.

Let's imagine together a few possible scenarios here. Because unplanned pregnancy is a pretty common thing, (otherwise most of us might not even be here right now, right?) it merits considering. Right now we are talking about this from the perspective of our parents, but maybe you have had a surprise pregnancy. The process is usually pretty similar, so let's talk this out.

Mom notices her period is late. She kinda wonders if she might be pregnant. And what is she thinking?

"Oh my goodness! We can't afford another baby."

"Oh no! Our other baby is just 3 months old! They would only be a year apart! I don't know if I can do it!"

"What? I just lost all my baby weight from my last pregnancy."

"But, I'm up for a big promotion at work ..."

"How will I finish college with a baby?"

"We just got married! We won't have any time to ourselves before our family comes along."

"My 'baby' is 14 years old. I'm not sure about starting all over!"

And you know, every time a mom discovers she is pregnant with multiple babies, there is a moment of "oh have mercy! TWINS?! How in the world will I keep up with two?!" It isn't that she's rejecting them, but there's a pretty strong emotional reaction, and yes, that may have a longer term effect on the babies.

This thought may only briefly flit across mom's mind. But, for a split second, the already growing baby inside may sense a twinge of rejection. Do you agree that this is a possibility? If not, the rest of this chapter will be a stretch for you, but don't cheat yourself out of the great stuff to come! Read on to discover some other possibilities, even if this is a bit "far out" for you.

So, if the baby senses a twinge of rejection at that point, does that rejection just go away after mom and dad realize how very excited they are about the new life growing inside her? I don't think so. But does that rejection affect the baby beyond the womb? Quite possibly.

In these scenarios, we are assuming mom quickly becomes excited about her new baby and the rest of the pregnancy is a breeze. But, what about morning sickness? What about other things that happen in mom's life during the remainder of the pregnancy? I truly believe that baby is picking up on way more than we tend to think and I'll share with you a bit from my own personal experience.

About three months before I became pregnant with my daughter, my dad was diagnosed with a terminal illness. The entire time I was pregnant, my dad was dying. He died when Bailey was 8 months old. If you have ever walked through terminal illness with a loved one, you know the roller coaster of events that you zoom through at speeds you couldn't have previously imagined. The races to the hospital in the middle of the night, hoping and praying you get there before he dies. Hoping you will get to tell him one last time you love him. The months of watching your "Superman" daddy become weaker and weaker. The deep feelings of grief and dreading a loss you can't imagine.

Do you think any of those intense emotions affected Bailey while she was in the womb? I didn't give that much thought at all. I was surviving the most difficult season I had walked through in my life thus far. Yes, I was comforted by my faith and yet I grieved so very deeply that I was losing someone I loved so much ... all the while growing someone I could not have imagined I could love so much. Talk about a paradox! It was that whole "best of times, worst of times" thing. So, did it have an effect on my unborn daughter?

Fast forward ahead about three years after she was born. One evening she was in the bath and I was hanging out nearby while she soaked and played in the bubbles. I don't recall if it was the anniversary of my dad's death, Fathers' Day, or any special date at all. But that evening I was feeling sad and missing my dad. You know how that can just bubble up without warning?

Bailey, being the observant person she has always been, quickly noticed I had tears in my eyes and yes, at the age of three asked me what was wrong. I told her "Oh baby, nothing's wrong. I'm just missing my daddy tonight." At that moment, she burst into tears herself. I was shocked. I asked her what was wrong. She said, "I miss your daddy, too." Then the waterworks were released! Her level of grief transcended anything I would have expected from a three year old who was only around her granddad for the first eight months of her life. She seemed grief-stricken. It was unreal to me. But at that point, I began to consider the possibility that she must have experienced some of my grief before she was even born.

Let's keep cruising. At this point you are either totally tracking with me, or you aren't. But whether rejection scts a seed while in the womb or not, it can set up camp at any other point during our lifetimes; and when it does ... it can wreak havoc.

When you were in school, did you ever feel "left out" from the rest of the group? Did you feel like there must be something about you that caused others to not want to let you be a part of them? That was rejection.

Did a high school boyfriend break up with you? Do you remember feeling rejected?

At work, do you ever feel like your coworkers are talking about you behind your back? Rejection strikes again.

How about at church? Does it seem like everyone else is operating on a higher spiritual plane than you do? Does it feel like you are missing out on something? Does it ever seem like maybe God loves someone else more than he loves you? Rejection! Rejection! Rejection!

What memory are you having right now in which you felt rejected? Write it down.

Take a moment to recall the feelings you felt when you were rejected. What were they? Loss? Grief? Confusion? Like you were less than someone else wanted you to be? Maybe you felt like you just couldn't be enough? Write that down here.

Looking back, can you see a lie from the enemy in that situation? Did you believe his lie over God's truth?

Now, let's pray and get the Holy Spirit's perspective on that situation.

Holy Spirit, forgive me for believing the lie that (name the specific lie you believed). I purpose and choose to forgive myself for believing this lie. In the name of Jesus, I cancel Satan's authority over me in this situation because it is forgiven. Holy Spirit, heal my heart and show me the truth about this situation.

Listen. Write down what the Holy Spirit just showed you about the rejection you felt.

You may have a difficult time recalling past rejection or even feeling its sting because you have already given forgiveness for that situation earlier in this book. It's essential we address past hurts, bitterness, and unforgiveness before we can dig into dealing with past rejection. If nothing is ringing a bell with you at this point, let's keep moving on. The Holy Spirit may bring up something a bit further along.

Let's switch gears from our feelings of rejection from other people to one that is even more biting, in my opinion. This is where we reject ourselves.

Self-rejection can be categorical, in which case we seem to reject everything about ourselves, often as a result of some self-unforgiveness, but this categorical self-rejection could be tied to receiving rejection from another person, too. And self-rejection can be specific, in which we reject specific qualities or facets about ourselves. Once we have consciously or subconsciously rejected ourselves in any way, it may open us up to receiving rejection from others, and/or even to acting in ways that attract rejection from others.

There's a crazy thing about rejection. Once we sense rejection from one person, it can cause us to act in ways that actually create rejection from others. It's as if we've received a rejection "brand" on our lives, and we may perceive that others reject us, even when they really don't. If we don't receive the rejection from them that we expect to receive, we may act in a certain way that causes them to reject us, either categorically or specifically. And while this rejection is very uncomfortable, it is oddly familiar.

While this is likely a new concept to you, I suspect you may be able to recall an example or two of someone acting in an unlovely way and creating a rejection against themselves.

One example I think of, having two sisters who have fostered and adopted children and having worked in child abuse investigation and reconciliation myself, is in the case of a foster child. He has been removed from a home where he wasn't safe. He's young and pretty confused about the events that have just taken place. Sure, the home he was in was neither comfortable nor safe, but it was familiar. It was painful, but familiar. And it's likely that by being removed from the home, he feels like his parents have rejected him. You may have strong opinions about child abuse, I think most of us do, but I truly believe that in most cases, the offending parent truly loves the child. Abusive parents have nearly always been abused as children themselves. Abuse, as ugly and painful as it is, is familiar. It may be all they know and the child may receive rejection (real or perceived) from the biological parent either before, during, or after being removed from the home.

So when the child is introduced into a new home, with new parents and new siblings, it is not at all uncommon that the child will act out in a way that may cause him to be rejected by anyone in the new home. At least if he's done something to cause them to reject him, the rejection won't be a surprise, nor will it be as painful as he may believe at some unconscious level. And while it is very uncomfortable, even the rejection is familiar.

You may not have been a foster child, you may have never encountered a foster child, but there are plenty of people all around you every single day who are suffering from the pain of rejection. Perhaps it was rejection from a severed relationship, from a job separation, from a move across the country, or even all the above. And when someone feels the sting of rejection, then they begin to act in ways that perpetuate the sting, it is difficult to find freedom from it until it is recognized.

As you read this, you may be realizing some rejection in your own life that you had not previously seen as such. You may be thinking about some old situations in a new light. As you go through your day today and tomorrow, you may be shocked by some of the words that come out of your own mouth and by the words you hear come out of the mouths of those around you.

It's my prayer as I write this that once again the Holy Spirit will reveal truth about this situation to you. I pray that He will gently bring to your awareness all rejection you have experienced, are experiencing, and any rejection that you are placing on anyone in your sphere of influence. By now you know He is gentle, but unyielding. He desires complete freedom for you. He doesn't reject you in any way, and He desires that you release rejection in every area of your life ... well, except for the righteous rejection of sin. The righteous rejection of sin is the only "good" kind of rejection I can think of. Otherwise, it's time to release rejection and embrace acceptance. Accepting yourself, in spite of the flaws you may have rejected for years, is a gateway to a fresh peace that you know you've been desiring in your life for a long time.

Releasing rejection and choosing to accept others is another key to restoring peace in relationships at home, at work, and in our communities.

Consider making a list of ways you have rejected yourself. Make a separate list for the ways you have rejected others. Ask the Holy Spirit to bring to mind every time rejection has reared its ugly head in your life up to this point and from this point on.

Pray through each individual rejection situation like this: *Heavenly Father, please forgive me for (this specific way) I have rejected (myself/ someone else). I purpose and choose to forgive myself for this situation and I cancel the enemy's authority over me in it because it is forgiven. Holy Spirit, show me the truth about this situation and heal my heart.*

As always, I suggest you write down what the Holy Spirit shows you after you pray. It's an ongoing source of encouragement and building up of my faith to look back on the ways He has revealed Himself and truth to me after I have prayed through situations. I want this same strengthening for you. Don't cheat yourself out of it by thinking you don't have the time. You are worth it.

Chapter Twelve

Have A Happy Ending

Have you enjoyed a deep, belly-jiggling, goofy-looking, ugly-snorting, laugh today? If not, did you get one in yesterday? I know, this is a pretty big subject change from last chapter's rejection topic, but isn't every book supposed to have a happy ending? The Bible certainly does!

I don't know about you, but I love a happy ending. I've been known on many occasions to flip to the back of the book just to see how it ends. I enjoy the stories more when I know how they end. It's okay to have a personal preference, right?

And who doesn't love to laugh! Oh, it may or may not be pretty, or sound graceful, or even be appropriate, but laughter is good medicine. If it's been too long since I had a good belly-jiggler, I'll find a movie or look at a book that gets me going, (Awkward Family Photos is my most proven laughter-giving book to date) or recount a hilarious and often-embarrassing story from the past with a friend or family member. Any one of these is sure to tip over my giggle box.

In his book, *Anatomy of an Illness*, writer Norman Cousins shared his personal story of overcoming serious illness and dealing with pain by watching funny television shows and laughing. He reported that, by belly laughing for 10 minutes, he could stave off the pain from the disease he was fighting for about two hours. Laughter is good medicine. Cousins also reported on several centenarians who were not only surprisingly old (one possibly as old as 150 years) but were described as spry, nimble, *and of good humor*. Laughter may not only be good medicine, but may be an important ingredient in a long life.

In Proverbs 17:22 we read, "A cheerful heart is good medicine, but a broken spirit saps a person's strength." (KJV) King Solomon, in all his wisdom, had discovered that laughter and being cheerful is good for one's health. So not laughing, or having a broken spirit, sucks the strength right out of us.

In Proverbs 15:13 we read, "A joyful heart makes a cheerful face, but with a heartache comes depression." (Names of God Bible) Doesn't everyone want a cheerful face? Sure we do! Doesn't a cheerful face have a more youthful appearance? You bet it does. And with all the money spent on face creams, lotions, potions, gels, and masks in hopes of appearing more youthful, why not take a few minutes each day to get in a good laugh? It's good for the spirit, soul and body, and it makes for a cheerful and youthful face.

What makes YOU laugh? How long has it been since your last belly-jiggling laughing fit? Maybe it's time to schedule some time to lighten your spirit and laugh a little – or a lot! And personally, I most enjoy laughing when I'm surrounded by family or friends. Oh sure, there have been plenty of times when I giggle or even full-on belly laugh when I'm alone (often provoked to such by something funny one of my beloved pets has done), but for some reason, like so many things, laughter is more fun with a friend!

Do yourself a favor and don't go to bed until you've had at least one good belly laugh every day for a week. Laughing at bedtime will relax your body, uplift your mind and emotions, and in my experience, set you up for a delightful night's sleep. Will you take the 7-Day Belly Laugh Challenge? And why not invite someone to take it with you? You might even learn a few good jokes from the whole thing!

Putting it all together. A day in the life of your Healthy Body.

As we wrap up our time together in this Healthy Body book, I thought it would be good to not only get you laughing, but to walk through a day in the life of a Healthy Body. It's my hope that the next few pages will share some practical applications for many of the health keys shared in this book. As you read this example, I hope you will see your new, free Healthy Body self in every paragraph.

Frankly, if I'd read this ten years ago or so, I would have thought to myself, "That's just totally unrealistic! No one can be that chirpy and happy all the time." But I typed much of this from my own personal experiences and yes, as I reviewed it one last time before sending it off for publishing, I got tears of joy in my eyes. I bless the

Lord for His healing work in my life. I bless the Lord for His healing touch in YOUR life. He is good. He loves us so immensely. He woos and pursues us and when we sense peace, it's His Shalom peace.

So let's start in the morning and wrap up with a happy ending!

Upon awakening, you take a few minutes to breathe deeply and thank God for blessing your life with another day. No matter the weather outside, today is always a beautiful day. There are beautiful people in your world, and you get up looking for, listening for, and expecting beauty and blessing.

Before you head out for a morning walk (and within 30 minutes of waking), you whip up a protein drink with at least 30 grams of protein to replenish the amino acids your body used in its housekeeping last night as you slept. You also swig down a glass of water to begin to replenish what was lost during respiration as you slept. That's important because you know you're always a little bit dehydrated upon awakening. Lots has gone on in your body since you conked out 8 hours ago or so.

During your morning walk you're recalling some of the blessings you've noticed over the past 24 hours. "Oh Lord," you think to yourself (or maybe you say it out loud), "thank you for my family. And especially for that sweet daughter of mine. Father, give her direction today. Attract her to your light and repel her from the ways of darkness that surround her." "Thank you for my husband. For the loving, hard-working man you've blessed into my life." "Thank you for this dog who's on-guard during our walk together. I love his companionship and the funny things he does that bring laughter and joy into my life." "Show me opportunities today to share your love with someone through encouraging them." "Thank you, Lord, for your creation. You are awesome! I love you, Abba Father!" You notice the flowers that are blooming today, but you didn't even notice their plants yesterday. You may see a new kind of bird, hear a new bird song you haven't noticed before, or even feel an extra pep in your step. Yes, you are especially chirpy, so far, today! What a positive start to your morning!

As you get back into the house, you notice someone has left some breakfast dishes on the table. Oh sure, that person (who doesn't really need to be named here, does he?) knows at some level that the dishwasher is dirty and "receiving" as we say in our house. But maybe he was busy thinking about sales reports, shipping, mowing the lawn, feeding the horses, ordering flea treatment for the cats, or a long list of other possibilities. And at this very moment, you have a choice to make. Will you bear offense because he didn't put the dishes up? Will you let this small infraction ruin your morning? Will this be the deal breaker of deal breakers for harmony in that relationship (at least for the next 10 minutes or so)? OR, will you purpose and choose to forgive, forsaking a right to offense, and as I used to say early in my marriage, "put those dishes up to the glory of Jesus?" You choose to forgive. The nameless person wasn't really attacking you. He was likely preoccupied. It's not a big deal – unless you make it one. But you're a quick forgiver now, so forgive quickly and move on. You're having a great morning, remember?

After you take the 35 seconds to put the dishes into the dishwasher while simultaneously praying through a forgiveness prayer for the dish-offender, you hop into the shower, resuming your attitude of gratitude for the blessings in your life. When you hop out, as you're wrapping up a quick skin brushing, you notice a text from your mom. She asks you to call her because she got some results back from the doctor. You instantly begin to feel the familiar pressure in your throat or chest area; it's fear. You notice your thoughts immediately wander to old familiar phrases, "Oh no! It can't be good. If it were good, she would have said so in the text. Oh no! What if it's cancer? What if I lose her? What if ..." But, before your what ifs continue, you recognize exactly what they are: they are harbingers of the old spirit of fear. You recognize its ugly "fingerprints" in this situation and you decide you will not go there. No sirree. You are so over coming into agreement with fear.

You speak aloud your favorite fear verse, 2 Timothy 1:7, to remind yourself that fear doesn't come from God. "For God has not given me a spirit of fear, but of power, love and a sound mind." Then you say aloud, "In the name of Jesus, I command the spirit of fear to go, now." Because NOW you know your authority. You are a co-heir with Jesus Christ, the son of God. NOW you know how to take care of some business. NOW you are free from the spirit of fear. You are walking in the spirit of truth and peace. So you do what you need to do, you call your mom back, and you experience a peace that passes understanding as she shares with you next steps in her medical process. You're no longer fearful. You are peaceful, which blesses you, and the spirit of peace is experienced by your mom and others. Bless the Lord.

After you get off the phone with your mom, it's time to head to the office. Your mind whirs with all the things you need to do today. Oh man, if only the boss could be out today. You could get so much more work done if she could work at a different branch today. And the co-workers...well, you used to feel like you didn't fit in. You felt like they didn't like you, but you didn't know why. After working through rejections in your life, God has shown you the truth. That you may not have a lot in common with them, but you've been put there for a reason. You are not rejected, but you are called to a higher purpose. And, as you've reached out to your coworkers, you've discovered that each one of them has some really beautiful qualities you couldn't see before.

By lunch time you are famished. A couple coworkers invite you to lunch at a yummy Mexican restaurant. Alright, you're strong. You can and you WILL make a Healthy Body choice when it comes time to order. You skip the chips, order fajitas with extra veggies, skip the rice and beans, order a side of guacamole and lettuce, then pour a small boat load of salsa all over everything else you're eating. It is delicious! You leave feeling not overly-stuffed like you have in the past, but comfortably satisfied and mentally sharp for the afternoon's activities. No carb-coma in your cubie today! Plus, you feel pretty doggone proud of yourself for blessing your body, not giving in to food choices that would lead to guilt, or even indigestion.

On your way back to the office, a car pulls out in front of yours and narrowly misses your front bumper. You quickly hit the brakes to avoid a collision and your co-workers try out some new names for the poor soul whose village is missing...someone... Okay, not really, but it's a scary event and once again, you have a choice to make. Will you waste some time and a lot of mental/emotional energy getting caught up in replaying the event over and over, only to make yourself madder and madder? Or will you quickly forgive the other driver, and choose to use words that are a blessing? I know it's counterintuitive at first, but over time I've trained myself to utter a quick prayer for that other driver, "Oh Lord, please keep them and others safe as they zoom along their way." There, so you've forgiven and chosen to speak a blessing. It's a double winner! Breathe.

This afternoon, you have a coaching session with an employee who's been underperforming. Sometimes it seems like she simply doesn't care at all whether or not her work is done right, or even at all. It can be frustrating to work through the process with her to give her every opportunity to succeed. Part of you wishes you could terminate her employment today, but you believe she has better in her, and you're willing to give her a chance to discover that. So, you use the power of your words during the coaching session to be honest and direct about the specific underperforming issues, but you also let her know you see better in her.

You speak in faith that you know she can do better. You remind her of the "wins" she's had in her position before. You ask her how she can help you see more of that than what she's been producing recently. You give her clear expectations, set a date for following up on her performance, and speak excellence into her. She leaves the meeting feeling challenged to do better, and knowing you believe in her. You leave the meeting relieved that it's over and knowing that you took the high road. Holding her accountable isn't being "mean." It's working with her in truth and helping her become more effective in her position. It serves everyone well.

Finally, the work day is complete and you head home. Tonight is flurry scurry. Your daughter has dance and your son has soccer. Your husband is handling dinner before everyone runs off in their own directions. During a quick dinner around the table, you take time to listen to the events of each person's day. Your daughter is struggling with math. You speak affirming words that encourage her that she has the mind of Christ. You let her know you believe in her. You tell her she's smarter than she knows. Then, it's divide and conquer as you hit the road!

While waiting at your daughter's dance practice, you notice another mom who has recently lost weight. You resist the old temptation to compare yourself to her. You resist the old habits of beating up on yourself because you may be a size or two larger than she is. Since you love yourself and have started making some gradual changes, your own habits will lead you to your healthiest weight and size. You're okay with that. You're happy for the other mom. And you're inspired to stick to your new health disciplines.

After everyone gets home, gets homework done, and starts getting ready for bed, you take a few minutes, maybe even sipping some hot tea, to reconnect with your tribe. This doesn't have to be an overly-structured time, but taking even 15-20 minutes to hear more about today, and getting a game plan for tomorrow, helps everyone feel valued and prepared for the day ahead.

After bedtime prayers and tuck-ins, you catch a soaking bath, curl up with a good book, and enjoy some time with your husband. Before you drift off to sleep, you take a few deep breaths, thank God for your blessings, and then drift off to sleep. You fall asleep quickly because you are at peace. You are relaxed. You've put in a good day's work and tonight you will sleep like a happy baby. You'll awaken refreshed tomorrow. Peace is on you. Health is in you. Joy surrounds you. You are a Healthy Body. Be blessed!

About DiAnna

DiAnna Wallace is a Naturopathic Doctor, Master Herbalist, Loomis Digestive Health Specialist, Certified Nutritionist, and Certified Natural Health Professional. She has a bachelor's degree in Psychology and homeschooled her daughter for ten years. She has practiced health consulting since 2007.

DiAnna is passionate about sharing health-giving, life-enhancing principles for every person, believer or not. Everyone desires better health, healthier relationships, and pain relief from a lifetime of hurts. DiAnna has demonstrated dogged tenacity by digging in with those she serves to help them get breakthrough and healing, not just for their bodies, but all the way to the molecular level. Only the Holy Spirit can bring this kind of molecular healing, and it is DiAnna's honor and joy to partner with Him in her work every day.

To find out how to have DiAnna speak to your group or congregation, visit www.diannawallace.com.

Made in the USA
Columbia, SC
06 May 2019